God's Healing Belongs 2 U

by

Nick Watson

I0222958

Nick Watson Prophetic Power Ministries

youcanprophesy@gmail.com

www.youcanprophesy.com

YouTube channel – https://goo.gl/U7L22u

God's Healing Belongs 2 U

ISBN-13: 978-0-9943012-5-3

Published by Nick Watson Prophetic Power Ministries.

Brisbane. Australia. 4178

DEDICATION

My four dedications of this book are:

- To the Lord Who has partnered with me in many ways to write it.

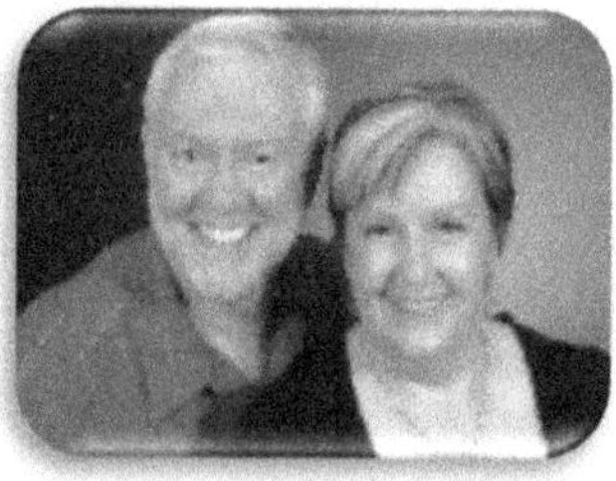

- To my wife Lynne and our family of four generations.

- To the healing ministers who have helped me grow in faith and ministry, especially the Lord Jesus Christ, and godly men and women who have shared their teachings, testimonies and tears in various Christian media, including the internet.

- To the people who will receive their healings through these teachings and testimonies and to those who will minister healing forward to others.

Author's Introduction

If anyone had told me years ago, that one day I would write a book on Divine healing, I would have laughed as Abraham (Genesis 17:17) and Sarah (Genesis 18:12) did. I spent many frustrated years in ministry because not enough people were being Divinely healed, despite what the Bible said about God being so very willing to heal all who come to Him through faith in the Lord Jesus Christ and in the Word of God, the Bible.

One day I got the revelation from the Word and Holy Spirit that if I wanted a healing ministry I had to turn my negative frustration into a positive desperation. Jesus' words in John 7:37-19 came alive to me. If I was thirsty for a Holy Spirit healing ministry I had to come to Him, not wait for Him to come to me, and take the healing anointing by faith.

So, for a year or more, I set my wide-ranging Bible reading aside and limited my reading to the Gospels and the Book of Acts. I bought, borrowed or watched online every healing teaching and testimony series I could. The result was that God showed me things by His Spirit and I learned and grew in faith for Divine healing. As I spent time in prayer, praise, worship and waiting on God, He changed me and my theology and imparted to me the faith and spiritual gifts I sought from Him. One of those spiritual gifts was the gift of healing pain and all its causes. While I cannot say everyone I pray for who is in pain receives a complete, permanent healing, I can say that in every meeting people are healed. Praise God, because only the Lord can heal anyone of anything. Praise Him also because He can heal everyone of everything! Hallelujah.

The greatest revelation I received was that healing is in the atonement. This means that when Jesus went to the Cross, He did so for both the forgiveness of our sins and the healing of our bodies (and the wholeness or shalom of our souls). So, if we can believe that our healings are fully paid for already, then we should be able to take by faith the gifts of individual, specific healings Jesus has made available for us to receive.

I believe people will be healed as they read this book. This is my prayer for you, my reader.

I believe people will minister healing to others as they grow in faith by reading this book. This is my prayer for you.

I give all the glory to Jesus for what has happened and will happen in healing ministry in and through my life.

ACKNOWLEDGEMENTS

I thank my amazing wife and the love of my life, Lynne, for being my indispensable partner in life and in ministry. Lynne was also my proof-reader.

I thank my editor-in-chief, John MacFarlane, without whose skills and efforts this book would not have come into reality.

Special mention and gratitude goes to Lisa Watson of the Printing Well, Wynnum for her sensational design of my book covers and other printing help she donated towards this project. ***www.theprintingwell.com.au/***

AUTHOR'S CHOICE

I have made two non-traditional choices in this book. Firstly, I have deleted the definite article "the" from the Name of Holy Spirit, because I want Him to become more personal to my readers. Secondly, I have capitalised a lot of pronouns (such as "Him"), in order to give the Lord the honour He is due and to make clear Who the pronoun represents.

BIBLE QUOTATIONS

Unless stated otherwise, all Bible quotations in this book are taken from:

Other versions quoted:

King James Version. Public Domain.

The Amplified Bible. Zondervan Bible Publishers. © 1965. 24th reprinting – April, 1982

The Jerusalem Bible. DARTON, LONGMAN and TODD Ltd. And Doubleday and Company. London. 1968.

Table of Contents

1 Jesus paid for your healing

Many of the testimonies quoted at the start of each chapter and others are available to view on my YouTube channel **https://goo.gl/U7L22u** They have also been uploaded to my Facebook page: https://www.facebook.com/nickjwatson.ycp

In time, new testimonies will be available on my Facebook ministry page: **Nick Watson Prophetic Power Ministries** and my website: www.youcanprophesy.com

Testimony

David came to the meeting in Atlanta, Georgia, USA with his hand and fingers frozen into a ball. It was as if he had been carrying an invisible baseball or tennis ball in his hand for the last 5 years. He'd had four surgeries that included having a metal plate inserted in his wrist. In one prayer, the Lord loosed him and restored full movement to all five fingers. Similarly, his hand and wrist were freed to function fully and

freely. How happy he was. His mouth was filled with praise. He could resume a normal life, using both his hands and all his fingers. Hallelujah.

> ... the punishment that brought us peace ("shalom") was upon Him and by His wounds we are healed.
>
> *Isaiah 53:5b NIV*

The broad meaning of "salvation"

Too many Christians have narrowed the meaning of salvation to only its spiritual dimension. They immediately only think of salvation as representing their reconciliation to God through the forgiveness of sins and faith in the sacrifice and triumph of Jesus. They limit salvation to the truth that they are now born again and Heaven-bound. However, a study of both the Old and New Testaments reveals that the Hebrew and Greek words, which in English represent salvation, are much broader in meaning. The words include concepts of rescue, being set free, provision, healing, restoration and victory. In other words, salvation is representative of a new relationship and partnership with God that impacts every area of our lives, including our spirit, soul, body, relationships, circumstances, finances, vocation and calling.

So, when you think of the word salvation in regard to what Jesus did for you, it is important that you understand "it's not just pie in the sky when you die; it's also steak on your plate while you wait." In other words, Jesus not only purchased eternal life in heaven for us who believe, but He also paid for us to enjoy an abundant life on earth. (John 10:10).

Christians must train their minds to think of salvation in whole-of-life terms, not just in the spiritual sense of being saved and therefore having a home in heaven. Narrow thinking in regard to salvation can rob us of faith for the many other benefits Jesus purchased for us by His suffering, sacrifice and triumph over sin, death and the devil. (read, for example, Psalm 103:1-5).

Don't think that God cares about you spiritually more than He does in regard to the quality of your earthly life. Such thinking will limit your faith to receive the whole-of-life benefits, including physical healing, that belong to you, because of Jesus.

The broad meaning of "shalom"

In Isaiah 53:5, the Hebrew word "shalom" is declared to be one of the benefits of salvation.

A quick internet study of the meaning of "shalom" will inform you that it is another whole-of-life word. It incorporates qualities such as wholeness, completeness, soundness, well-being, prosperity, security, tranquillity and orderliness. Some have summarised it by this phrase: "nothing missing; nothing broken."

"Shalom" includes peace with God in our spirit; the peace of God within, that is, in our soul, our inner being, our mind, will and emotions; peace and good health in our body; peace in our relationships and circumstances; peace that comes from victory over opposition and adversity; peace in our finances; peace in our ministries for the Lord.

So, when you think of the word 'shalom–peace' in regard to what Jesus did for you, you must train your mind to automatically believe that Jesus was punished so you could receive God's peace in every area of your life, including physical healing.

Often when I am ministering, especially if I am preaching in regard to Isaiah 53:5, I will get the congregation to say the following out loud after me – and I encourage you to do this now, as you are reading this page:

Jesus got what we deserved, which was punishment .... So that we would get what He deserves, which is blessing, peace and healing. "

Jesus paid for your healing.

Theologians would echo this by saying "Healing is in the Atonement". If you can get a revelation of this Biblical fact, your healing will soon appear.

Remember Who wrote the Bible. It is not the writers whose names are associated with the different books that make up our Bible. The true Author is Holy Spirit Himself.

You will see His Divine Hand as we consider the following passage.

> 4 Surely he has borne (nasa) our sicknesses (choli) and suffered (sabal) our pain (makob): and we considered *him stricken, smitten of God, and cast down. 5 But he was wounded for our rebellions; he was bruised for our iniquities; the chastisement (punishment) of our peace was upon him; and by his stripes (wounds) healing was provided for us. 6 All we like sheep have become lost; we have turned each one to his own way; and the LORD transposed in him the iniquity of us all.*
>
> *Isaiah 53:4–6 JUB*

In the construction of these three verses, Holy Spirit has deliberately intertwined twin themes regarding our salvation, namely, the forgiveness of our sins and the healing of our bodies.

In verse 4a, He writes about the physical healing of our bodily sicknesses, weaknesses, malfunctions, breakages and pains. In verses 4b and 5a, He refers to the forgiving of our sins and the removal of both the penalty and power of sin, by the Blood of Jesus.

In verse 5b, Holy Spirit returns to the physical and soul-realm aspects of our whole-of-life salvation.

In verse 6, He goes back to the spiritual dimension of our salvation.

This style of writing deliberately unites, in an inseparable way, the concept that Jesus' suffering, sacrifice and triumph purchased for believers both their forgiveness and healing.

Some of the translators tried to "spiritualise" or "emotionalise" the Hebrew words "choli" and "makob" in Isaiah 53:4a. They moved away from the physical nature of the meaning of these two words and used spiritual or emotional words like griefs and sorrows.

Holy Spirit made clear these words were to retain their primarily physical meaning when He wrote Matthew 8:16-17 into the Gospel record.

> *16 When evening came, many who were demon-possessed were brought to him, and he drove out the spirits with a word and healed all the sick. 17 This was to fulfill what was spoken through the prophet Isaiah: "He took up our infirmities and bore our diseases.*
>
> *Matthew 8:16-17 NIV*

To linguistically reinforce the point, Holy Spirit used the very same two Hebrew verbs ("nasa" and "sabal") found in Isaiah 53 verse 4a again in verses 11 and 12. By so doing He was telling us again, in a subtle way, that the very same actions which Jesus did in his passion were designed to both purchase healing for our bodies (in verse 4a), and the forgiveness of all our iniquities and sins (in verses 11 and 12).

This twin aspect of our salvation is confirmed elsewhere in the Bible, notably, in Psalm 103:3, James 5:14–16, 1 Peter 2:24 and in the account of the forgiveness and healing of the paralysed man, who had four friends. (Mark 2:1–12).

One can also see both the forgiveness of sin and the healing of the body in the account of Moses raising up the bronze serpent in the wilderness. The incident is recorded in Numbers 21:4–9. In John 3:14, Jesus explained the incident was a foreshadowing of His crucifixion and our salvation. Again, we must conclude that Jesus' sacrifice on the cross and His triumphant resurrection were for both our spiritual salvation and physical healing.

We must understand that Jesus was punished twice. Many criminals would have been mocked and scourged and then sent home. Jesus was both scourged and crucified. Wounding His Body was sufficient for our physical healing; but Jesus had to die, as did the animals in the Old Testament sacrifices, in order for our sins to be forgiven and for us to receive the righteousness of God.

Here is the most important consequence of believing this teaching: If you get a revelation from God, based on what and how Holy Spirit wrote about Jesus paying for both your physical healing and the forgiveness of your sin, then, just as you used your faith to receive your spiritual salvation, so you will be able to use your faith to receive your physical salvation, which is your healing.

Here is a one sentence summary of what this chapter means in regards to the healing aspect of your whole-of-life salvation and shalom: **Healing belongs to you because of Jesus**.

I encourage you to stop reading right now and say as a confession of your faith 3 times:

- Healing belongs to me because of Jesus
- Healing belongs to me because of Jesus
- Healing belongs to me because of Jesus

Let these Scriptures reinforce your faith confession: Romans 8:32; 1 Corinthians 3:22b–23

What is one thing you have learned from this teaching?

____

What is one thing you can do to implement this teaching?

____

Faith Declaration:

I thank You Lord for paying the price for my whole-of-life salvation. I praise You for not only forgiving my sins, so that I have eternal life, but also for granting me all that I need to have abundant life on earth. I thank You Jesus for paying the price for my inner and physical healings. I praise you for the fact that healing belongs to me, not because of my performance, but because of what You did for me and for all who believe the good news of the Gospel and the New Covenant. By faith, I receive my healing now, in Jesus' Name. I command my body to be well and every symptom of sickness, weakness and dysfunction to stop now for the glory of God, in Jesus' Name. Amen.

2 Why God heals

Testimony

Eddie came to the meeting in Dunoon, Scotland. Some years previously, he was in such a bad car accident that the emergency service first-responders had to cut him out of the car. He did not realise how badly he had injured his knee. Being a drug addict at the time, he did not feel any serious pain for quite a while so, he did not seek any medical treatment for it. His knee got worse and worse because he was working in the physically demanding landscaping industry. When Eddie did see the doctors an X-ray showed that his knee was shattered, with fractures like a spider's web. That night as Eddie put his faith in Jesus and tested out his knee, he felt the warmth of Holy Spirit activity in the knee for about 10 minutes. He was completely healed. He told me a couple of days later how he could do so many things without pain that had previously caused him trouble. He was full of praise for the Lord and had such a big smile on his face as I videoed his testimony. It is uploaded on my YouTube channel.

Awesomely, the next night in Greenoch, Scotland, Eddie's wife, Sharon, was healed of her lower back problem. Hallelujah. How great is our God.

Many people would like to think that God heals simply because someone has a need. Sadly, that is not true. This way of thinking is just as wrong as expecting the Lord to forgive every sin, without the need for any repentance or faith in Jesus' forgiveness.

The fact is that both forgiveness and healing are triggered by a person's faith in God and His Word to receive His spiritual and physical salvation.

I acknowledge there are four instances in the Gospels where Jesus was moved by compassion to heal needy people.

The first instance is Matthew 14:14. Jesus had compassion on the 5,000-plus people. He healed their sick, which is what many of them would have come to receive. My understanding is that both faith and compassion were operating in this instance.

In the second and third cases, Jesus was first asked to heal the person. (Matthew 20:24 and Mark 1:41). In other words, both faith and compassion were in operation.

The fourth miracle is the only one in which there is no recorded request nor any presumed expectation on behalf of the recipient to be healed. It is the resurrection of son of the widow of Nain from the dead.

My point is this: If you want to wait for the compassion of Jesus alone to receive your healing, without the need for anyone but Jesus to have faith, you could be waiting a very long time and your need would have to be very desperate indeed.

The reality is that God is moved by compassion, but He requires someone to have faith before healing is received.

If need alone was sufficient for healing to be manifest, there would not be a sick person in the global church, nor in all the nations, because it is clear from Jesus' ministry that the Lord has compassion for sinners as well as saints.

So why does God heal the sick?

(1) To demonstrate His Nature and fulfil His Covenant Name and Responsibilities

> ... I am the Lord Who heals you.
>
> *Exodus 15:26b NIV*

Firstly, God is absolutely committed to demonstrating Who He is. This is what sets Judeo-Christianity apart from other religions. God has revealed and continues to reveal Himself to us as the all-seeing, all-knowing, all-powerful, all-holy, all-loving Lord of all creation, which He made, He sustains and with which He communicates.

All other religions are man-made, not God-initiated. Their "gods" are blind, deaf, dumb and powerless, because they are mere imaginations, glorifications of other humans or demonic deceptions.

Healing, like Loving and Doing Good, is not just something God does, it is an expression of Who He is. God is Love; God is Good; God is Healing.

As Creator God, He made us in His Image and He put the DNA of healing into our bodies. Our bodies fight for the restoration of good health because this is the Nature of God in us.

Healing reveals God's Love, Compassion and Mercy. (Acts 10:38; Matthew 20:34).

Healing reveals God's Divine Authority and Power. (Luke 5:20-26; John 10:38; Exodus 15:26).

Secondly, God is absolutely committed to fulfilling His part of the New Covenant that He has sealed between Himself and His people by the Pure, Precious and Powerful Blood of Jesus. The Name Jehovah Raphe in Exodus 15:26, essentially means this: I am the Lord, to Whom nothing is impossible. I hereby commit Myself unconditionally (in the New Covenant; the context of the revelation of this Divine Name in the Old Testament was conditional) to be your Healer. I will heal you whenever you have a need. (But, we must have the faith to receive it). I will heal you because I have committed Myself to take the responsibility for your healing as My part of the Covenant between us.

(2) God Heals to honour His Son and the Name of Jesus

> *8 Being found in appearance as a man, He humbled Himself by becoming obedient to the point of death, even death on a cross. 9 For this reason also, God highly exalted Him, and bestowed on Him the name which is above every name, [10] so that at the name of Jesus every knee will bow, of those who are in heaven and on earth and under the earth, 11 and that every tongue will confess that Jesus Christ is Lord, to the glory of God the Father.*
>
> *Philippians 2:8–11*

Firstly, God heals in order to honour the price, the very highest price that has ever been or could ever be paid namely, that of the obedience of Jesus unto the point of death. Jesus paid for our full salvation. If God did not heal today, that would be like saying Jesus' sacrifice and triumph was not enough for everyone, for every need, for all time. However, we are assured that Jesus' once-for-all sacrifice and triumph is sufficient for every need of every person, in every nation and in every generation, by Bible verses such as Hebrews 9:11–15; 10:10; 10:14; 1 Peter 3:18; and 1 John 2:2.

In this regard, as you read these Scriptures about Jesus dying once for all, you must bear in mind, as you have seen in chapter 1, that our salvation includes both the forgiveness of our sins and the healing of our bodies.

Secondly, God wants to demonstrate that Jesus is not dead; rather Jesus is alive and He is Lord. In John 10:25; 10:38 and 14:11, Jesus said that if people didn't believe His words, they should believe in Him because of the miracles He did. This was because the evidence of the power and authority of God gave credence to Jesus' words.

It is still the same today. Miracles done today in Jesus' Name give credence to Jesus' words, as recorded in the New Testament, just like they did in the days following His resurrection and ascension to Heaven. (Acts 3:16-19; Acts 4:4,10,12,21). Miracles today demonstrate that Jesus is alive and that He is Lord!

Thirdly, healing demonstrates that the Name of Jesus is indeed the Name above all names. (Philippians 2:9). This includes names such as pain, cancer, sickness, arthritis, inflammation, displacement, deterioration and all other names of any and every debilitating problem in our lives. Hallelujah.

Some time ago, Holy Spirit revealed this to me: 7 things that happen when the Name of Jesus is spoken in faith and heard in the heavens.

(i) In the heavens, it sounds like 10,000 x 10,000 voices as angels respond in praise. Just as God amplified the footsteps of the four lepers in 2 Kings 7:5-6, so the Name of Jesus resounds throughout the heavens, like the sound of many waters or many huge Niagara-sized waterfalls. (Ezekiel 43:2; Revelation 1:15 and 19:6).

(ii) The Name of Jesus gets the Father's immediate attention. This is like any mother who hears her child laugh or cry; or like proud parents hearing their own child's name called out at a graduation ceremony.

(iii) Father God treats prayer in Jesus' Name as if Jesus Himself had prayed it, because Jesus is our Great High Priest. (Hebrews 4:14-16). If in the parable, the generous father said "yes" to his prodigal son, how much more will our Heavenly Father say "yes" to us. Father God would never refuse His own Son, Jesus, Who both intercedes for us and allows us to use His Name in prayer. That is just like our earthly fathers allowing us to use their credit cards to make purchases.

(iv) The Name of Jesus reminds God of the Covenant Price Jesus paid for those who pray in His Name. It reminds Father God that Jesus' Covenant Price has paid for all the blessings, victories and resources His followers need to succeed in life, godliness and ministry. These include full salvation, which means the Lord's whole of life partnership and "shalom" in every area of life. It also reminds the Father that Jesus has said "YES" to all the promises of God in His Word. (2 Corinthians 1:20). Note that for these promises to be fulfilled in our lives, we must say the Amen both in words and by faith actions.

(v) Jesus' Name means God Saves. This Name reminds Father God that He has work to do and it motivates Him to do all that Salvation includes and to release all the new covenant blessings and resources that are written in His Word.

(vi) Jesus' Name causes demons on earth and in the spirit realm to tremble and flee, because Jesus Christ is Lord.

(vii) Jesus' Name causes miracles to happen on earth because Jesus' Name is the Name above all names, including pain, injury, deterioration and disease. Jesus' Name is as ointment poured forth. (Song of Solomon 1:3 KJB; ESV). When we speak out the Name of Jesus we release both the power of Holy Spirit and the authority of the Most High God and His Champion and Captain, our King of kings and Lord of lords.

The Name of Jesus is also above the name of every demon that causes our problems. In Jesus' day, some people may have been healed of physical epilepsy caused by a physical accident of some kind. Others had to have a demon of epilepsy cast out of them. Similarly, some deafness problems are purely physical in nature; others are caused by demons.

This book is about physical healing, rather than deliverance.

(3) God Heals to honour His Word and to Fulfill His Will on Earth

> *So will My word be which goes forth from*
> *My mouth; It will not return to Me empty,*
> *Without accomplishing what I desire,*
> *And without succeeding in the matter for*
> *which I sent it.*
> *Isaiah 55:11 NASB*

God heals because "He cannot lie" (Hebrews 6:18 and Numbers 23:19). He cannot say "I am the Lord Who heals you" (Exodus 15:26b) and then refuse to do it. He cannot write in His Word that by the wounds of Jesus we are healed (Isaiah 53:5b) and then refuse to make that a reality in our lives. (refer Matthew 8:14-17).

God cannot make the promise that believers can lay hands on the sick and those sick people will get well, without backing up that promise with actual healings taking place. Those healings will be evidenced by Divine power, not just by the normal recovery process of the human body, nor only from what can be explained by medical means. (Mark 16:18b,20).

When Jesus taught us to pray "Your Kingdom come, Your Will be done on earth as it is in Heaven" (Matthew 6:10), He was declaring, in effect, that God wants to reproduce the conditions of Heaven on earth, just as He did in the Garden of Eden.

God's Healing Belongs 2 U

There is no sickness in Heaven. There was no sickness in Adam's domain on earth until the devil and sin came to our planet.

The intervention of Jesus into human affairs on earth has made it possible for all things to be restored to the way God ordained it and made it at the time of His Creation of all things. This includes a reversal of the dual curses of sin and sickness that have afflicted Adam's race. Hallelujah.

You must believe and be assured that it is God's Will for you and every human being to be healed and not sick.

What is one thing you have learned from this teaching?

What is one thing you can do to implement this teaching?

Faith Declaration:

I thank You Lord for healing me because You are true to Your Own Nature and to Your Word and to Your Son. I am grateful for and give You praise for Your Grace and Power. There is no-one and nothing too hard for You. You are faithful and powerful to perform all You have written in Your Word. Thank You Jesus for Your suffering and triumph on my behalf. By faith, I receive my healing now for the glory of God and the honour of my Lord and Saviour and Healer, Jesus Christ. I command the devil to flee from me and stay gone, in Jesus' Mighty Name. Amen. I command my body to be well and every symptom of sickness, weakness and dysfunction to stop now and never return, in Jesus' Name. Amen.

3 Faith is necessary to receive

Testimony

Jacquie came to Apostolic Churches of Canada annual convention in Montreal. She was in the meeting when I spoke about Holy Spirit and ministered healing to the sick. For six years, Jacquie had been taking pain-killers on a daily basis. She said she ate them like they were candy. Jacquie had tripped and fallen down a flight of stairs, badly injuring her lower back. As she stood in faith, she heard a "pop" while I was speaking the healing into being. She tested her back out and there was no pain from any movement she undertook. Eight days later, I was preaching at her local church in Peterborough. She told me she was praising God because He had given Jacquie her life back. She could walk, run, sit, lift and do anything without even a hint of pain. There was absolutely no restriction to her movements. Hallelujah!

As I said in Chapter 2, the reality is that having the need for a healing is not enough to guarantee that the Lord will heal you.

If need was enough to move the Hand of God, there would be no needs left to heal in the whole world. That's how loving and powerful He is. His healing is not reserved for special people, not even His Own people. His healing, like His spiritual salvation, is available for everyone.

But, like His spiritual salvation, His healing can only be imparted and received when someone has the faith to believe it will happen, before it happens.

> *And without faith it is impossible to please* Him, *for he who comes to God must believe that He is and* that *He is a rewarder of those who seek Him.*
>
> *Hebrews 11:6 NASB*

For healing to take place, someone must have the faith to receive it or minister it. Preferably both the healing minister and healing recipient believe, along with everyone else in the room.

> *For by grace you have been saved through faith; and that not of yourselves, it is the gift of God;*
>
> *Ephesians 2:8 NASB*

This verse declares a Divine principle that applies to everything we receive from God. As previously explained, salvation is a whole-of-life concept. Therefore, a Christian is:

- Saved by grace through faith
- Forgiven of their sins by grace through faith
- Cleansed from all unrighteousness by grace through faith
- Set free from the bondage and power of sin by grace through faith
- Healed by grace through faith
- Made whole by grace through faith
- Blessed by grace through faith
- Empowered by grace through faith

Every person who desires healing should ask to receive healing ministry from Christians who believe not only that God heals today, but that He will heal whoever asks for healing "in Jesus' Name". The asker has the right to expect that the minister believes this.

I found seven specific instances in the Gospels where Jesus credited a person's faith as the reason they experienced healing.

(1) The centurion (Matt.8:13)

(2) The woman who touched the hem of Jesus' garment (Matt.9:22)

(3) The 2 blind men (Matt.9:29)

(4) The Syrophonecian woman whose daughter was delivered (Matt.15:28)

(5) The four friends who brought their paralysed friend to Jesus (Mark 2:5)

(6) Blind Bartimaeus (Mark 10:52)

(7) The grateful, tenth leper (Luke 17:19)

Faith is a Forest, not a Mountain

Faith is not just a mysterious spiritual "thing" that you grow until you can say to someone: "my mountain of faith is bigger than your mountain." If there is even a grain of truth in such a statement, it is more likely that your small sand-castle of faith is bigger than his tiny faith ant-hill.

That kind of thinking is entirely wrong. Firstly, we should not ever compare ourselves with others.

Secondly, faith is something that has to be built in specific areas of life, so that every Christian has a strong tree of faith for each of the following:

(1) Knowing that they are saved and heaven-bound

(2) Holiness of lifestyle;

(3) Inner peace and strength;

(4) Physical healing;

(5) Positive relationships; and

(6) Finances that are sufficient to share with others;

(7) Ministry to others

(8) Etc. etc. etc.

If you want to be healed or to exercise a healing ministry, you must build your own faith to receive physical healing and to minister it to others. I speak from experience.

Over a two-or-more-year period, I focussed my Bible reading on the four Gospels and the Book of Acts. I bought many series of Christian Healing teachings. I watched YouTube testimonies and teachings about physical healing. Progressively my faith increased.

Of course, I prayed for the sick. Over a period of time, the number of people who were healed after I prayed for them "in Jesus' Name" increased.

> *..., Jesus stood and cried out, saying,* "If anyone is thirsty, let him come to Me and drink.
>
> *John 7:37*

In this verse, Jesus tells you that if you want anything from Him that you do not presently have, including sufficient faith, you must go to Him. You cannot simply wait and hope that He will come to you.

The Lord rewards those who diligently seek Him. If you want to be healed by God, you must take responsibility for growing your own faith.

If you want to have a ministry of healing for others in Jesus' Name and for His glory, you must take responsibility for growing your own faith.

One of the ways we grow our faith is by growing in our knowledge of God and His Word.

> *So then faith comes by hearing, and hearing by the word of God.*
>
> *Romans 10:17 NKJV*
>
> *.... those who know their God will be strong & do exploits*
> *Daniel 11:32b*
>
> *..... Call unto Me and I will answer you and show you (reveal and demonstrate to you) great and mighty things.*
> *Jeremiah 33:3*

What is one thing you have learned from this teaching?

___

What is one thing you can do to implement this teaching?

___

Faith Declaration:

I thank You Lord that when I put my faith on the line, You respond from Heaven. When I do what the Bible says, You do what the Bible says. I thank You that I can trust You to do miracles and to release Your provision in every area of my life. I praise Jesus for saying "Yes" to every promise of God in the Bible and for paying the price for them to be made available to me, as a joint-heir with Him. I say the "Amen" for both my own healing and wholeness and for my healing ministry to others. I command my body to be well and every symptom of sickness, weakness and dysfunction to cease now and never return, in Jesus' Name. I ask and believe for the Lord's health to be my portion throughout my life, as Jesus and Moses and others in the Bible demonstrate. I speak into being that when I minister to the sick they will be supernaturally restored to full health and well-being, in Jesus' Name. Amen.

4 Healing is God's Will

Testimony

In Chester Hill, Sydney, Pastor Chris Blackley had lots of pain issues right throughout his body because he had worked in the construction industry for years. In his video testimony, he said: "Glory to God, Who loves me and cares for me, because all my pain has gone. I am not the same; I am healed".

In Los Angeles, Pierre, the Youth Pastor of South Bay Celebration (AoG) church, had severe back pain for more than a week. He missed church the previous week because of it. Pierre came in faith on the Sunday I ministered there. He testified that, after I prayed for him, which was before church started, he was free of all pain. Ps. Pierre was able to fully enter into worship with no restrictions to his body movement.

> 40 And a leper came to Jesus, beseeching
> Him and falling on his knees before Him,
> and saying, "If You are willing, You can

> make me clean."[41] Moved with compassion, Jesus stretched out His hand and touched him, and *said to him, "I am willing; be cleansed."
>
> *Mark 2:40-41 NASB*

It is important to realise that, according to John 20:30-31, only a fraction of all the healings and miracles that Jesus did are included in the Gospels. The ones that have been included are designed to teach us something and build our faith.

The healing of the leper has a number of important lessons. For the sake of this section, I am going to call the leper by the name Jerry, which could be short for Jeremiah.

Lesson One: When you are sick, you must come to Jesus for healing. You are the leper who initiates your healing. You don't wait for God to heal you. In most of Jesus' healings, including this one, the Syrophonecian mother, the centurion's servant and the nobleman's son, the people came to Him to ask for healing. In a few cases, such as the healings at the Pool of Bethesda and in the village of Nain, He initiated the healing.

It is noteworthy that this is one of the instances of healing when Jesus was moved by compassion. However, His compassion was not stirred until the leper came to Him for healing!

Lesson Two: Don't let religious thinking stop you from getting healed by our Lord Jesus.

According to Deuteronomy 28:27and 59–61, the leper could have assumed his sickness was a punishment from God for his sins and disobedience to God's Word.

The leper, whom I am calling 'Jerry', could have thought, "God has willed my suffering, so I cannot be set free from it unless and until God heals me". If it really was God's Will for him to be sick, Jerry should not have sought either medical help, nor supernatural healing, for fear of doing something that displeased God.

The very fact that Jerry approached Jesus in this way indicates that firstly, He considered Jesus to be the Messiah, the One sent from God. Luke 5:12 tells us that Jerry called Jesus "Lord".; Secondly, he believed in the principle of Isaiah 40:1–2, namely, that he had suffered enough and it was time for the comfort of God to be given to him; Thirdly, he believed in the power, authority and goodness of God through His anointed and appointed Messiah, Jesus, in accordance with the promises of Isaiah 61:–2a. Perhaps Jerry had heard that Jesus quoted this as His job description in Luke 4:18–19.

Lesson Three: It was God's Will to heal Jerry. It is always God's Will to heal all who come to Him. God's Will is whatever promise or principle is in His Word.

> 14 This is the confidence which we have before Him, that, if we ask anything according to His will, He hears us. 15 And if

> we know that He hears us *in* whatever we ask, we know that we have the requests which we have asked from Him.
>
> *1 John 5:14–15 NASB*

There are four reasons why we know healing of the sick is always God's Will.

(1) Jesus perfectly revealed the Will of God. Jesus is the express image of God. (Hebrews 1:3; Colossians 1:15). Everything Jesus did showed us exactly what the Father is like and what His Will was and is. According to what Jesus said in John 5:19–20, everything Jesus did was by the specific leading of the Father. Jesus' entire ministry on earth was a perfect fulfilment of the Will of God. (John 5:30,36).

(2) Jesus unconditionally and completely healed every person who came to Him. Therefore, the example and teachings of Jesus tell us that it is the will of God for every person who comes to Jesus to be healed.

As I wrote in Chapter 1, healing is included in what Jesus did for us before, on and after the Cross. Because salvation is available to all it follows that healing is available to all.

(3) Jesus has said "yes" to every general and specific promise of God in the Bible, including those that directly relate to healing. 2 Corinthians 1:20 tells us that we must say the "Amen" or "so be it" in both words and deeds, in

order to receive our healing. It is our healing, not our sickness that is to the glory of God.

> *For no matter how many promises God has made, they are "Yes" in Christ. And so through him the "Amen" is spoken by us to the glory of God.*
>
> 2 Corinthians 1:20 NIV

(4) The fourth reason why we know that healing is God's Will is because Jesus treated all sickness as being the devil's work, not God's. 1 John 3:8 tells us that Jesus came to destroy the works of the devil, which include sin, sickness, poverty, injustice, soul-sickness, demonic oppression, depression and possession etc.

> *how God anointed Jesus of Nazareth with the Holy Spirit and power, and how he went around doing good and healing all who were under the power of the devil, because God was with him.*
> *Acts 10:38*

> *[11] and a woman was there who had been crippled by a spirit for eighteen years. She was bent over and could not straighten up at all. [12] When Jesus saw her, he called her forward and said to her, "Woman, you are set free from your infirmity." [13] Then he put his hands on her, and immediately she*

straightened up and praised God.....[16] Then should not this woman, a daughter of Abraham, whom Satan has kept bound for eighteen long years, be set free on the Sabbath day from what bound her?"
Luke 13: 11–13, 16

General promises about healing:

Psalm 34:10; Psalm 84:11; Matthew 7:7–12; John 14:13–14.

When you consider these general promises, you must have faith that "everyone" includes you; "whatever" includes your healing; "good things" and "good gifts" include your healing.

Specific promises about healing:

Isaiah 53:4–5; Psalm 103:3; Proverbs 3:7–8 and 4:20–22; Jeremiah 33:6; James 5:14–16; 1 Peter 2:24.

What is one thing you have learned from this teaching?

What is one thing you can do to implement this teaching?

Faith Declaration:

I thank You God for Your Grace by which you have made available to me so many benefits that are contained in the Gospel and purchased for me by the suffering, sacrifice and triumph of Your Divine Son Jesus, my Saviour, Healer, Provider and Lord. I praise You because I can confidently say: Healing belongs to me because of what Jesus did for me. Right now in Jesus' Name, I claim my healings and I command my body to come into line with the Word of God, and to serve the Lord and His purpose by serving me in fullness of bodily health and strength, in Jesus' Name. I command every affliction of the devil to be loosed from me now and permanently, in Jesus' Name. Amen.

5 Is healing unconditional? Yes and no

Testimony

Geoff came to his usual church in Market-Rasen, Lincolnshire, England one Sunday morning when I was the guest minister. He had undergone several operations on his hip, but still limped when he walked and had to use a cane to help ease his pain. That morning after just one prayer, Holy Spirit quickened his mortal body. People who had been in the church for years saw Geoff walk without a limp, without pain and without his cane. Two months later, the woman in the church who had organised with her pastor for me to minister that morning, visited Australia to see her family. Mary said Geoff was still doing extremely well. The Lord had done more for him through one prayer than doctors had been able do in various operations. How great is our God. Praise Him from Whom all blessings and all healings come.

> 4 I have brought you glory on earth by finishing the work you gave me to do.
>
> *John 17:4*

Part 1 – from God's perspective, the answer is "yes", healing is unconditional.

In the Gospels, Jesus never told a single person that they had to fulfil any condition before they could be healed. He never once said: "I can't heal you because God is not happy with your bad temper"; or "God told me that because you lied to your wife, you have to wait until next week to be healed"; or "You have been so sinful that God has told me to give you a bad knee to go with your migraine"; or "You can only be healed after you repent of theft and pay the money back to your boss, or your customers, or your neighbour."

From God's point of view, there are no conditions to be fulfilled for any person to be physically healed, because Jesus has fulfilled every covenant requirement for us.

Jesus said on the Cross: "It is finished". (John 19:30). Our salvation was fully paid for by what Jesus did. There is nothing more that has to be done by God for our sins to be forgiven or our souls restored or our bodies healed.

There is nothing we can add to what Jesus did for us. There is nothing we can do to "earn" or "deserve" our salvation. All I can do is to believe that what Jesus did is enough for my whole-of-life salvation and receive by faith what has been given to me unconditionally by the grace of God.

Jesus paid for every sin to be forgiven, every soul need to be met and every physical problem to be healed.

In order for my sins to be actually forgiven, 1 John 1:9 tells me that I have to confess my sins, as an act of faith in what Jesus has done for me. When I do so, God is faithful to forgive my sins and cleanse me from all unrighteousness. In other words, what Jesus paid for becomes a reality in my life after I believe that His sacrifice and triumph are enough for my need.

In order for my body to be healed, I have to have the faith to receive what Jesus has already done for me. "By His wounds, we are healed". (Isaiah 53:5 NIV). "By His wounds you were healed". (1 Peter 2:24b NASB). "By His wounds you have been healed". (1 Peter 2:24b NIV).

Again, I say that on God's side, there is no condition required for any human being to receive salvation or healing or any other Grace-given blessing or empowerment. Jesus has paid for all things.

God does not judge the sick person to see if they have been good enough to earn their healing or bad enough to not only be refused the healing Jesus has already given them, but also so bad that God might afflict them with more health and other problems.

You must know that because of Jesus, God has changed the way He deals with people. He hasn't changed His

Nature, but He has changed His "rules of engagement". God has changed the way He deals with us.

No longer does the Old Testament, as typified in Deuteronomy 28, apply. Under that system, if God's people were obedient, they were rewarded with many desirable blessings. If they were disobedient they were afflicted with all kinds of punishments, including sickness, poverty and defeat.

However, the New Testament's new Covenant of Grace means that God pours out His blessing on us unconditionally because of Jesus, not because of our performance. Hallelujah.

Part 2 – from man's perspective, the answer is "no", healing is not unconditional.

The one and only condition for us to receive healing is this: "Someone has to have faith". His, her or their faith is necessary for someone to receive the healing that belongs to us because of Jesus.

A good illustration of this is when Jesus went back to His own home-town of Nazareth.

> 5 *He (Jesus) could not do any miracles there, except lay His hands on a few sick people and heal them.* 6 *He was amazed at their lack of faith.*
>
> Mark 6:5-6 NIV

Think about the concept of Jesus not being able to do something He wanted to do. After He left the Cross, Jesus overcame death, as was prophesied about Him in Psalm 16:10. Jesus spent time in Hell, defeating the devil and publicly humiliating him and his demons. He also preached to and released various captives.

Finally, Jesus reclaimed the full authority over the earth that Adam had forfeited to Satan through his sin in the Garden of Eden.

If Jesus cannot be stopped from doing God's work in Hell, how can He be stopped on earth?

The correct understanding of Mark 6:5 is not that the unbelief of the Nazarenes prevented Jesus from doing His mighty works. Rather, the true interpretation is that their lack of faith hindered them from receiving the healings and miracles that Jesus could have done, if they believed in Him.

The following verse confirms my interpretation of Mark 6:5 and shows you just how necessary faith is.

> 2 *For indeed we have had good news preached to us, just as they also; but the word they heard did not profit them, because it was not united by faith in those who heard.*
>
> *Hebrews 4:2 NASB*

The possessing of the Promised Land in the Old Testament is an example of how faith must be used to receive the blessings God gives us by Grace. In Joshua 1 verses 2 and 3, God says He is giving the land to the Jews, but their feet must tread on their inheritance. In other words, the land will only become their possession when they go into it and conquer its inhabitants and begin to farm it for the harvests it will bring them.

In healing ministry, we have to fight by faith against all the symptoms, diagnoses, doubts, fears, criticisms, unbelief and demons that stand against us. Because the battle is the Lord's and Jesus has already won the victory, we can be successful in making our promised inheritance of healing a reality in our lives... even if it takes a big battle or a lot of wrestling to see it fulfilled. Israel had to fight 3 battles in order to conquer the land, so let us fight with courage and persistence for our healing and for a healing ministry to others. (Joshua 1:6–9). God will never deny you the miracles you need because He has already punished His Son so that you can have God's Peace in every area of your life. By Jesus' wounds, you are healed. (Isaiah 53:5).

Focus your thoughts and words on Who Jesus is and what He has done for you. Jesus got what we deserved, which is punishment, so that we could get what He deserves, which is blessing. Hallelujah. Keep acting in faith, as Israel did, and you will surely possess the healings Jesus has purchased for you. Remember, healing belongs to you, just as every other blessing of salvation does, because of Jesus, not because of your performance, nor because you are trying to earn or deserve it. You must receive every promise of God, every Grace-blessing by faith

The reality of the power of both God and faith is revealed in these two verses.

> *For nothing will be impossible with God.*
>
> *Luke 1:37 NASB*

> *And Jesus said to him, "... All things are possible to him who believes."*
>
> *Mark 9:23 NASB*

These verses show us that our faith can draw every heavenly blessing and resource to earth to meet even impossible needs. Mind you, the fact that faith makes impossible things possible, does not mean that having faith makes impossible things easy. There can be work to do before a miracle is manifest. That is why the spiritual gift in 1 Corinthians 12:10 is called the "working" or "energising" of miracles.

We must build our faith as a lifestyle in order to be ready for the moment when miracle-working faith is needed. No-one can live a life of wishy-washy faith or faith that constantly flirts with doubt and fear and think they will be used by God to bring about miracles in times of great or urgent need.

Holy Spirit does quicken the spiritual gift of faith to Christians in tough situations, but always He releases the gift to those believers who put their faith on the line day-in and day-out, in every area of life. As a comparison, Holy Spirit will not give the gift of discerning of spirits to someone who is a negative-minded, tearing-down-others, self-righteous, critical person. He will look for someone humble, but strong, with a good knowledge of God's Word, a commitment to righteousness, truth and justice that is balanced with a loving approach to people.

There is another line of thought about having faith that is based upon Mark 11:22. Young's Literal translation brings out the Greek meaning that we can "have the faith of God", whereas other versions use the expression "have faith in God." We can ask God to impart His perfect, problem-solving, miracle-working faith to us. Again, I believe God would do that if we are already using our own faith as a lifestyle. The Lord's compassion could motivate Him to give a dose of His faith when a believer is faced with a problem where people are distraught. An example would be when a child is struck with a serious sickness. The apostle Peter may have been given the Lord's faith or the Holy Spirit's spiritual gift of faith when he was used to raise Dorcas from the dead in Acts 10:40.

The Church's problem is not limited to the fact that many Christians lack faith and therefore need to do the spiritual things that are necessary to build their faith in order to both receive healing and minister healing to others.

According to Jesus in John 10:10, there is a spiritual thief who wants to rob us not only of what we have, but also of what we should have, because it is part of our inheritance in Christ. Therefore, Christians must develop their spiritual discernment and strength. One of the key ways our enemy the devil does his evil thieving and destroying work is to take our focus away from Jesus. Stop looking at yourself and your problems and symptoms. That depletes your faith. Fix your eyes on Jesus and the Word of God and your faith will grow and your healing will come.

Our other problem, aided by wrong teaching in the Church and by demonic deception, is that we think there are lots of conditions to be fulfilled before we can be healed. Such thinking prevents us from using our faith to receive the healing that belongs to us, because of Jesus.

- We think that if we "feel unworthy", God won't heal us. We do not receive anything from God based upon our feelings. Everything we receive from God comes to us because we believe what the Bible says. The fact is that we are made worthy in Christ and by Christ.

One of the most important lessons we learn from Isaiah 53:4–5 and the Gospel of Grace in the New Testament is this: "Jesus got what we deserved, which is punishment, so that we could get what He deserves, which is blessing." Hallelujah!

- We think that if we haven't "performed" morally or religiously or spiritually well enough, God won't heal us. The reality is that our healing has already been purchased for us, based upon Jesus' performance. It is not at all dependent on our performance. Jesus is still willing to heal both saints and sinners alike.

Our self-righteous, self-condemnation blocks us from receiving our healing just as happened (for different reasons, but with the same result) in Jesus' hometown. Our own negative attitudes rob us of faith, multiply our doubts and build a barrier of unbelief that prevents the blessings of God from flowing into our lives, just as surely as an umbrella stops the refreshing rain from falling on us.

In Acts 13:46, Paul told the Jews that because they considered themselves unworthy of the blessings and benefits of the Gospel, he was going to preach instead to the Gentiles. The Jews missed out on God's salvation, favour, power, healing and blessing because of wrong attitudes that they could have changed. Please do not make the same mistake they did. Consider yourself a candidate for healing because God loves you and Jesus paid the price for your healing. Trust God. Believe in Jesus and the promises of God's Word. Act in faith according to the Divine promises and you will receive your healing.

What is one thing you have learned from this teaching?

___

What is one thing you can do to implement this teaching?

___

Faith Declaration:

Dear God I am so grateful for what You did for me. Thank You for sending Jesus. Thank You Jesus that You came, You suffered and You triumphed for me and for all who believe in You and the Word of God. Thank You for qualifying me, who is so unqualified in myself, to be a co-heir with You. Thank You Father for graciously giving me, along with Jesus, all things, including my healing. (Romans 8:32). I praise You for being Jehovah Rapha, the Lord my Healer. I take authority over my mind, my feelings and every demonic deception, in Jesus' Name. I bring every thought captive and into alignment with God's Word. I thank You Lord that I am worthy in Christ and I receive my healing by faith, in Jesus' Name. Amen. "

6 Two major blockages to healing

Testimony

In Augusta, a lady pastor came to the meeting at Grace Place. She had years of problems with severe dry eyes. She awoke 2 or 3 times every night to apply more gel. That process was uncomfortable, being much worse than using simple eye drops. As I ministered the prayer of faith, she felt the cool, living waters of Holy Spirit washing her eyes. She felt instant relief. She called me a couple of days later to say she was sleeping all through the night, which was a wonderful testimony on its own, and that her eyes were perfectly normal. Hallelujah!

14 For if you forgive others their trespasses [their reckless and willful sins], your heavenly Father will also forgive you. 15 But if you do not forgive others [nurturing your hurt and anger with

> *the result that it interferes with your* relationship with God], then your Father will not forgive your trespasses.
>
> *Matthew 6:14–15 AMPL*

Unforgiveness

Unforgiveness is the greatest and most common hindrance to people receiving their healing. It is not the case that their refusal to forgive prevents God from making real in their body the healing Jesus has already given them. Rather, their feelings of anger, bitterness, revenge, hurt and offence pollute their soul and they do not feel worthy of being healed. Some people actually feel they should be punished for their negativity or for some sin they have committed.

While it is true that the prayers of the unforgiving person are hindered, that is not true of the person who is ministering healing to them. So, healing can still flow. However, the healing may only be partial and could prove to be only temporary.

The real problem is that the receiver is blocked by his own negativity and by the accusations of our enemy the devil, who takes advantage of the situation.

Virtually every major healing minister and ministry has testimonies of people receiving their physical healing as soon as they let go of their unforgiveness and associated negativity. There are lots of instances where arthritis has been healed. As I was writing this book, I met Chuck from

Lincolnton, South Carolina. He had a work accident that resulted in him having several operations on his foot. Over a period of more than four years, doctors were puzzled as to why his healing was not happening. One night the Lord woke Chuck up in the very early hours and said "You will not heal until you forgive the boss of the company that did you wrong regarding the accident." Chuck obediently went to the company office and apologised for all the hatred that had built up in his heart toward the man. Chuck thanked him for the good employment he had experienced there over the years. The boss was literally speechless and just sat there with an open jaw. Chuck's healing kick-started that day and was soon complete.

Of course, the best thing to do for your own inner peace, health and strength is to forgive others quickly. You do this by faith, not by emotions. Only after you forgive will you be healed within. When you have a healthy soul, you will be more able to exercise your faith to receive the healing of your body.

I must make reference to the situation between husbands and wives, and indeed between all family members. It is hard to forgive and keep on forgiving when the offences come thick and fast on a regular basis. However, by faith we must persist in following the principles of God's Word, even up to 70 times 7 occasions ...... and that could be per month or week or even day ! (Matthew 18:21-22).

> *Similarly, you husbands should try to understand the wives you live with, honouring them as physically weaker yet equally heirs with you of the grace of eternal life. If you don't do this, you will find it impossible to pray properly.*
>
> *1 Peter 3:7 Phillips*

Remember three things:

- If you don't forgive, you hinder your own healings in your soul and physically. Choosing to not obey God in this matter becomes the sin of disobedience, or, what is even worse, rebellion. Never forget that sin lets the devil in. He wants to make your life miserable and worse than it is now. Don't give him that opportunity. He can turn any small foothold into a stronghold of negativity in your life.... and he will, if you let him. Light and darkness do not dwell together. Holy Spirit is grieved by our sin and will not abide in darkness. What He wants is our invitation and faith to evict sin, darkness, depression, fear, anger, bitterness, sickness and every evil thing from our lives.

- Love covers a multitude of sins. (Proverbs 10:12; 1 Peter 4:8). So, keep on loving your family and even your critics, opponents and enemies, by faith. This will help you have a healthy soul and a healthy body.

Over the years, I have been hurt many times. I have learned the hard way how to forgive by faith and how to be healed inside.

I have had to forgive some people of the same, single major thing a thousand times. I have had to ask God for healing a thousand times. I discovered one sure way to be healed inside. That way is to ask God to bless those who hurt you.

I don't mean ask God to bless them by sending a lightning bolt to torch their new Mercedes in order for them to realise how arrogant they are. I mean ask God to give them every blessing you desire for yourself and your family and future.

Another vital aspect of becoming free and healed and at peace is that we must remove our judgement from those we consider have done us wrong. Let God be their Judge.

- As I wrote in my book *34 Faith-Lifters*, you must also forgive yourself for sins you have committed and mistakes you have made and problems you have caused for others.

An Unhealthy Soul

> *Beloved, I pray that in all respects you may prosper and be in good health, just as your soul prospers.*
>
> *3 John 2 NASB*

This prayer works in reverse, that is, in the negative, as well as in the positive. If you have a healthy soul, this will have a good effect on your body and lifestyle and circumstances. If you have an unhealthy soul, this will have a negative impact, as doctors will tell you, on your physical health, and on your relationships, including your relationship and partnership with God, your finances and other areas of your life.

Understand that the soul comprises our mind, both conscious and sub-conscious, our will and our emotions. Any of these areas can be unhealthy, and they interact, so unhealthy emotions can lead to unhealthy thinking and unhealthy decision making and vice versa.

Our conscience is another dimension of our spirit and soul. This too must be kept holy in order to be healthy.

> *[21] Dear friends, if our hearts do not condemn us, we have confidence before God [22] and receive from him anything we ask, because we keep his commands and do what pleases him*
> *1 John 3:21-22*

Some signs of an unhealthy soul are found in the following Bible verses.

> *All the days of the despondent and afflicted are made evil [by anxious thoughts and foreboding], but he who has a*

glad heart has a continual feast [regardless of circumstances].

Proverbs 15:15 AMPL

5 Those who let themselves be controlled by their lower natures live only to please themselves, but those who follow after the Holy Spirit find themselves doing those things that please God. 6 Following after the Holy Spirit leads to life and peace, but following after the old nature leads to death 7 because the old sinful nature within us is against God.

Romans 5:5–7a

We demolish arguments and every pretension that sets itself up against the knowledge of God, and we take captive every thought to make it obedient to Christ.

2 Corinthians 10:5 NIV

For God did not give us a spirit of timidity or cowardice or fear, but [He has given us a spirit] of power and of love and of sound judgment and personal discipline [abilities that result in a calm, well-balanced mind and self-control]

2 Timothy 1:7 AMPL

Having a healthy soul involves overcoming all the negativity that the devil, the world, people and your own sinful nature throw at you. It really is a battle, a battle we can surely win if we let Jesus be truly Lord of the whole of our lives and if we renew our minds by and in accordance with the Word of God.

We must do things God's way, in the power of Holy Spirit, in order to overcome the relentless onslaught of negativity that affects our minds, emotions and choices.

It takes deliberate, consistent effort to develop and maintain a healthy soul.

It has been described as a battle because:

(1) Your mind does not want to give up control of your life to the Lord;

(2) The devil will not cooperate with you as you seek to shut out his influences, which include lies, accusations, temptation, discouragement, depression, oppression, and condemnation. He knows that he will lose his control over you, once you learn to consistently choose right, holy, positive thoughts and reject wrong, sinful, negative ones; and

(3) We are constantly subjected to negative influences from people in our lives and from various media.

Through faith and persistence, the Lord will help you, by His Word and Holy Spirit, to overcome bad mental habits.

You will break free of controlling influences such as fear, worry, anger, poverty, guilt, lust, greed, inferiority, inadequacy, depression and pride. You will live a new and better life.

Here are some things you can do to have a healthy soul

- The greatest key to having a healthy soul is knowing who you are in Christ, knowing the overwhelming oceanic love and mercy God has for you personally and knowing that the grace of God is super-abundant and unconditional toward you, because it is based on Jesus' performance, not yours.
- Take the time and make the effort to renew and retrain your mind, especially by the Word of God. You cannot think negatively all the time and live a positive life.
- Be sanctified in spirit, soul and body.
- Be healed of your hurts.
- Let go of your offences and unforgiveness.
- Repent of your sins and the offences you cause others to experience.
- Get control of your emotions. This is not an easy thing to do, but it is necessary.
- Get control of your tongue. This is not an easy thing to do, but it is necessary.
- Get whatever help you need.

- Exercise self-control, in all areas including your finances and your tongue.
- Command the devil to "get the hell out of your head"
- Seek more joy in your life.

> *A cheerful heart is good medicine, but a broken spirit saps a person's strength.*
> *Proverbs 17:22 NLT*

> *Finally, brothers, whatever is true, whatever is noble, whatever is right, whatever is pure, whatever is lovely, whatever is admirable – if anything is excellent or praiseworthy – think about such things.*
>
> *Philippians 4:8 NIV*
>
> *For as he thinks within himself, so he is.*
>
> *Proverbs 23:7b*

No-one can have both a positive life and a negative mind and mouth. Right thinking leads to victorious Christian living. Stinking thinking leads to mediocrity, negativity, frustration and failure.

Positive Christian thoughts are full of faith, hope, love, wisdom & holiness. Negative thoughts are full of fear, doubt, confusion, guilt, depression, anger, inadequacy, hopelessness, envy, resentment and unforgiveness.

All the days of the afflicted are bad,
But a glad heart has a continual feast
[regardless of the circumstances].
Proverbs 15:15 (Amp)

For many years, I had an unhealthy soul because of weaknesses in my inherited DNA, a dysfunctional only-child upbringing and a lack of knowledge as to how to handle life and do life.

When I came to the Lord, I wanted to get healthy and strong inside so I could live a positive life that I could both enjoy and use for the glory of God and the benefit of people in my world.

It took lots of years of absorbing God's Word to get close to God, to learn His ways, to accept my new identity in Christ and to allow His Indwelling Holy Spirit to overcome my natural negativity and build faith that overcame my pessimism and fear.

I know from personal experience that having a healthy soul will help you receive answers to prayer, including healings and miracles, from God.

Again, I say that the greatest key to having a healthy soul is to be overwhelmed by the infinite, unfailing and unconditional love of God. Bathing constantly in His love and His unearned grace and undeserved favour washes away all the junk and rubbish that accumulates in our hearts and minds. You feel clean, refreshed and strong. Hallelujah.

What is one thing you have learned from this teaching?

____

What is one thing you can do to implement this teaching?

____

Faith Declaration:

I thank You Lord for giving me new life, as a child of God, within and without. I am so grateful that You have given me a full inheritance in Christ including health, well-being and abundant life. Thank You for giving me Your Word to renew my mind and remove the offences I have harboured inside. By faith I now forgive those who have hurt me, including .... *(insert specific names here).* Thank You for giving me Your Spirit to restore my soul and heal my hurts. Lord I ask You to cleanse and heal my mind and heart afresh right now. Search me O God and see if there be any wicked or unworthy way in me. Create in me a clean and pure heart O God and renew a right and steadfast spirit within me. As I hand over my hurts to You for healing and yield my offences to You for forgiveness and a change of attitude, I also believe for my physical healing to be manifest now and I declare it will be so, in Jesus' Mighty Name and for His glory. Amen. Lord I declare Your protection over me to shield me from receiving hurts and offences. I declare that I have Your Holy Spirit inside me empowering me to not over-react to such things. I thank You that I have Your love, wisdom and strength to overcome all negativity and to not cause hurt or offence to others, in Jesus' Name. Amen.

7 Defeating doubts

Testimony

Courtney came to the meeting believing for the healing of a digestive problem she had endured for a long time. It was related to lactose intolerance and involved bloating and discomfort. Her life was restricted in regards to diet and still she experienced these uncomfortable symptoms. At the time of healing prayer ministry, she felt instant relief from all symptoms. As soon as she could after the ministry time, Courtney went to the kitchen and drank a full glass of full cream milk. I would never have advised her to take such a dramatic step of faith. I would have agreed to her taking a couple of small mouthfuls. She knew her healing would be for real. If it wasn't, she would be very uncomfortable, very soon.

Courtney returned for the night meeting totally healed of both the digestive problems and the lactose allergy. Hallelujah.

In a small meeting in Scotland, a mother and son moved their knees and legs in faith. They were both healed. Donald's mother was virtually dancing around the hall, after years of knee pain and restricted movements. Donald himself was facing a physical test by the local Fire Department the next morning. He came to church desiring a healing so he wouldn't lose that position. God met him and he was pain-free with full mobility.

> [22] *And Jesus *answered saying to them, "Have faith in God.* [23] *Truly I say to you, whoever says to this mountain, 'Be taken up and cast into the sea,' and does not doubt in his heart, but believes that what he says is going to happen, it will be* granted *him.* [24] *Therefore I say to you, all things for which you pray and ask, believe that you have received them, and they will be* granted *you.*
>
> *Mark 11:22-24*

The first tactic the devil used in the Garden of Eden to trick Adam and Eve into sinning and losing both their inheritance and authority was to plant the seed of doubt in their minds. (Genesis 3:1).

From there Satan progressed to a direct contradiction of God's Word (Genesis 3:4) and slander against the Lord's character. (Genesis 3:5).

This illustrates the danger of entertaining doubts. They grow to where you disbelieve the promises of God and even begin to feel negative about Him Who is perfect in Himself and in all His ways.

There is a difference between having doubts in your heart and mind. The Scripture in Mark 11:23 talks about not having doubts in your heart. You get rid of heart-doubts by building strong Biblical conviction within, that the Word of God is true, that God is good and great, that Jesus is Lord, that Holy Spirit is always with you and for you, no matter what!

Doubts of the mind are like the famous old saying about temptation: "You can't stop a bird from flying overhead; but you can stop it from nesting in your hair."

You get rid of mind-doubts by learning the Bible and choosing to replace your negative thoughts with the positive truths of God's Word. You train yourself to doubt your doubts and feed your faith.

Jesus said to the apostle Thomas: "Stop doubting and believe." (John 20:27).

If Jesus said it, then it is possible to do it, that is, to stop doubting and to believe instead of doubt.

Jesus connected doubt and fear by the following two statements:

When Peter began to sink after walking on water toward Jesus, the Lord said:

> *"You of little faith," He said, "why did you doubt?"*
>
> *Matthew 14:31 NIV*

When the disciples feared their boat would sink during the storm while Jesus was asleep, the Lord arose, rebuked the storm and the winds and waves became completely calm. He said:

> *"You of little faith, why are you so afraid?"*
>
> *Matthew 8:26 NIV*

It is also possible to stop fearing and believe.

When David fought Goliath, the whole Israelite army was paralysed by fear. David was in exactly the same position as they were, but he chose faith instead of fear.

From David's experience and other Biblical examples, including Gideon, Holy Spirit taught me this saying:

Every situation of fear is also an opportunity for faith.

The way to overcome both doubts and fear is by choosing what God says in His Word above all else. You must choose to evict all doubts and fears and replace them with the plain statements and promises of God in the Bible.

There are two keys to doing this. The first is to be a consistent reader, student and doer of God's Word.

> *31 So Jesus was saying to those Jews who*
> *had believed Him, "If you continue in My*
> *word, then you are truly disciples of*
> *Mine; 32 and you will know the truth,*

> *and the truth will make you free."*
> *John 8:31–32 NASB*

A lifestyle of continuously absorbing and acting upon God's Word will fill your mind and heart with faith that will overcome all your doubts and fears. You will come to choose the faith option, as readily as you choose to answer "four" when someone asks you the question: "What is two plus two?"

This is not to say you will never have doubts. When doubts come, you will have the spiritual strength to rebuke them and focus on the promises of God, drawing faith for your miracle from them.

Neither does it mean you will never experience fear. Like Gideon, however, you will be able to confront your fears and overcome them. Just as we resist the devil until he flees from us, so we must resist the fear until it is evicted from our mind and emotions.

There is something else you can do to overcome fear.

> I sought the Lord, and He answered me,
> and delivered me from all my fears.
>
> *Psalm 34:4 NASB*

According to 2 Corinthians 10:5 you must take captive every thought to make it obedient to Christ and the Word of God.

Discipline yourself to not continually focus on your symptoms, because that will feed your doubts and fears. Discipline yourself to meditate on God's Word, because that will inspire your faith and lead to life, peace, health, victory and prosperity.

There will be certain areas where you have really built your faith with the Word of God. When the enemy attacks you with doubts or fear, you will unhesitatingly choose what God says. That's when you know a miracle is on its way to you.

Jesus' brother warned us that like oil and water, doubt and faith do not mix.

> 6 *But when you ask, you must believe and not doubt, because the one who doubts is like a wave of the sea, blown and tossed by the wind. 7 That person should not expect to receive anything from the Lord.*
>
> *James 1:6–7 NIV*

Here are some common doubts that you must overcome:

(1) "God does not treat all people the same, so He might have helped others but I doubt He will help me." This attitude is false because the Bible says God regards favouritism as a bad thing. (Romans 2:11; Proverbs 24:23; 1 Timothy 5:21; James 2:1). Both the leper who asked Jesus if He was willing to heal him and the father who said "Lord, I believe, help my unbelief" believed Jesus could

do anything but doubted if He would do it for them. They had trouble exercising their faith for their own, personal need. You must overcome such doubts. You are a child of God, a co-heir with Christ. Healing belongs to you because of Jesus. You are included in all the "everyone" and "whatever" verses in the Gospels.

Over the years, I have been impressed by something Jesus said 5 times in just three consecutive chapters in the Gospel of John.

These verses indicate three things

(a) the infinite power, authority and resources of God;

(b) His limitless generosity and grace;
and

(c) the universal nature of His covenant commitment to His people to provide not only for all our needs, but for all we need to succeed, and to supply not just the barest sufficiency but as much as an overflowing supply. (Psalm 23:5; 2 Corinthians 9:8; Ephesians 1:3; Philippians 4:19; Hebrews 13:21; 2 Peter 1:3)

As you read these 7 verses in the Gospel of John, notice the fourteen (14) times Jesus said "you". He meant both "you" today, and "you" being the people who were with Him at the time. So, in Christ you, my reader, are a beneficiary of these promises, which include your healing. You are not excluded from any of the promises of God.

Notice also the words I have highlighted in bold print "whatever" (4 times), anyone and anything. These sayings of Jesus should ignite your faith for many answers to prayer in your life, for matters that are both small and big, and urgent, important and/or desirable.

> *Truthfully,* ***anyone*** *who has faith in Me will do what I have been doing. He will do even greater things ..... And I will do* ***whatever*** *you ask in My Name, so that the Son may bring glory to the Father. You may ask Me for* ***anything*** *in My Name and I will do it.*
> *John 14:12–14*

> *If you remain in Me and My words remain in you, ask* ***whatever*** *you wish and it will be given to you. This is to My Father's glory, that you bear much fruit, showing yourselves to be My disciples.*
> *John 15:7–8*

> *You did not choose Me but I chose you and appointed you to go and bear fruit – fruit that will last. Then the Father will give you* ***whatever*** *you ask in My Name.*
> *John 15:16*

> *..... Truly, truly, I say to you, **whatever** you ask of the Father in my name, He will give it to you.*
> *John 16:23 ESV*

(2) “I am getting old and can’t expect to be healed, because degeneration is normal for everyone.” Moses (Deuteronomy 34:7) and Caleb (Joshua 14:10–11) would disagree! So does the Bible in Psalm 103:5, which says God will satisfy your desire (for healing) and renew your youth.

(3) “Maybe it’s not God’s Will or time for me to be healed. Maybe He has a good purpose to be fulfilled during my sickness.” You must believe that just as Jesus healed all who came to Him, unconditionally and in the “now” of their need, so He will do for you. It is always God’s time to heal people, including you. There is no Biblical, New Covenant basis for thinking that God uses sickness to bless or teach people any good thing, especially His Own people. The Lord treated all sickness as a curse and work of the devil and never as a gift from, or teaching instrument of, or punishment from God. (Acts 10:38).

(4) “I don’t have enough faith to receive my healing.” Deal with your doubts and any fear you have regarding your problem and simply use the faith you have. Just a

mustard seed size of faith that is not mixed with doubt, fear and unbelief, is enough to miraculously move mountains of negativity.

(5) "I don't deserve my healing." Maybe you feel unworthy. Maybe you caused the problem. These things do not matter to God. Just as you would do everything you could for your child, regardless of their behaviour, so will the Lord do for you. God, your Father, has good gifts and Holy Spirit ministry for all His children. (Matthew 7:11; Luke 11:13).

What is one thing you have learned from this teaching?

____

What is one thing you can do to implement this teaching?

____

Faith Declaration:

I thank You Lord for enabling me to grow from faith to faith, strength to strength, glory to glory, victory to victory, anointing to anointing, healing to healing and blessing to blessing. By faith I take authority over doubts in my mind and over the spirit of fear that affects me from time to time. I bring every thought captive to the obedience of Christ. By faith I speak the truth of God's Word over my life and my body. In Jesus' name I declare I am of good health in my soul and therefore in my body and life's circumstances. I receive my healing by faith, because God's Word says that by Jesus' wounds I am healed. I command my body to be well and every symptom of sickness, weakness and dysfunction to leave me now and never return, in Jesus' Name. Amen.

8 How God Heals part one

Testimony

When I ministered in a church in Edinburgh, Scotland, the Pastor's personal assistant was healed. She had daily pain in both her feet for eight years. During the prayer ministry time, she released her faith to receive the healing that belonged to her because of Jesus. By the evening, she testified to the Pastor that she was healed and had been pain free all afternoon.

When you are seeking a healing from God, you need to understand that there are a variety of ways through which you can obtain that healing. If one way doesn't work for you, be persistent in seeking your manifest healing. That could be by continuing with the same healing strategy a number of times or by employing another of God's healing strategies. In fact you can express your faith through more than one of the Lord's healing methods simultaneously. The key thing is: keep believing and don't give up until you are healed.

Remember that faith is the key to receiving every blessing, healing and resource from God that His Grace has made available to you through the life, suffering, sacrifice and triumph of Jesus.

Maintain your faith in God's Character (such as His faithfulness, willingness and goodness), God's Word (including His promises of and principles concerning healing), God's Power and the Authority of the Name of Jesus, the Name above all names (including the names of pain, sickness, degeneration, injury, demons etc.).

How does God Heal?

(1) By His Word

> [20]My son, give attention to my words; Incline your ear to my sayings. [21] Do not let them depart from your sight; Keep them in the midst of your heart. [22] For they are life to those who find them and *health* to all their body.
>
> Proverbs 4:20–23 NASB
>
> He sent His word and healed them,
>
> *Psalm 107:20a*

The most famous Gospel illustration of this is found in the great faith of the centurion who asked Jesus to heal his sick servant.

> *[8] The centurion replied, "Lord, I do not deserve to have you come under my roof. But just say the word, and my servant will be healed..... [13] Then Jesus said to the centurion, "Go! Let it be done just as you believed it would." And his servant was healed at that moment.*
> *Matthew 8:8,13 NIV*

Here are five ways to receive healing through the Word of God:

- Reading the Word and listening to sermons helps you to "forget not" who you are in Christ and what you are entitled to because you are in covenant relationship with the Lord God All-Mighty. (Psalm 103:1-3).

- Hearing the Word – including when you speak it out loud to yourself – stimulates your faith to receive your healing. (Romans 10:17).

- Meditating on the Word causes you to be prosperous and successful. (Joshua 1:8). The two Hebrew words used in this verse literally mean (a) to make wise decisions (including about your health); and (b) to advance against the enemy and against opposition. This means getting victory over sickness, both spiritually, mentally, emotionally and physically.

- Speaking the Word releases the power of God to perform the Word, just as it did in Genesis chapter 1, and releases Holy Spirit to do His miraculous works, as happened in the valley of dry, dead, defeated, disconnected, destitute bones in Ezekiel 37. Holy Spirit was hovering over the problem until God's Word was spoken. Speaking the Word shifted Holy Spirit from atmosphere to action. When you speak the Word of God over your situations, it releases Holy Spirit to enact the Word of God and bring manifestation of it into the reality of your life.

> *For as many as are the promises of God, in Christ they are [all answered] "Yes." So through Him we say our "Amen" to the glory of God.*
> *2 Corinthians 1:20 AMPL*

This verse says that if we choose to speak in agreement with the promises of God, then He will be glorified. How will God be glorified (in the context of this book)? By our healing and by the healings we minister to others.

You must understand how powerful you are in Christ and how powerful your God-aligned words are. When you speak God's Words, you release Holy Spirit to do good things and good things happen.

If you choose to not speak in accordance with God's Word, then the promises of God will probably remain nothing more than a spiritual theory in your life. You will be frustrated, because things are not happening in your life. You may start blaming God in your heart, thinking He does not care for you or that His Word does not work for you. The truth is that if you do not speak or act in accordance with God's Word, then there is no guarantee that His covenant promises or any good prophecies you have received will ever come to fruition in your life. We need to co-operate with God and put our faith into action. One way of doing this is by speaking out the promises of God in His Word.

> *The tongue can bring death or life; those who love to talk will reap the consequences.*
>
> *Proverbs 18:21*

Our words can help or hinder our healing. Don't be constantly rehearsing your symptoms, problems and fears to yourself or others. Speak words of life, health, hope and faith. God will reward those words with the fulfilment of what you are speaking and believing. (Proverbs 12:14 and 18:20).

Job 22:28 affirms the power of decreeing the Word of God.

> *"You will also decide and decree a thing, and it will be established for you; and the light [of God's favour] will shine upon your ways.*
>
> *Job 22:28 AMPL*

The Hebrew word translated as "established" literally means to "arise, stand up". What you say will become a reality in your life. If you say something in agreement with God's Word, the Lord will do it.

One of the greatest lessons Holy Spirit has taught me is this: "When Christians do what the Bible says, God will do what the Bible says."

So, keep speaking God's blessing over your body, your mind, your life, your family, your finances, your future and your ministry. (Numbers 6:22–27).

- Preaching the Word releases the Power of God.

Signs and wonders, including healings follow the preaching of the Word.

> *20 Then the disciples went out and preached everywhere, and the Lord worked with them and confirmed his word by the signs that accompanied it.*
> *Mark 16:20 NIV*

(2) Laying On Of Hands

According to Hebrews 6:2, this is a "foundational" doctrine and ministry. Therefore, every believer should know about and use the ministry of Laying On Of Hands.

This ministry (which I will abbreviate here as "LOOH") occurs when a Christian places his or her hand(s) in faith upon someone, believing for the recipient to experience physical and/or inner healing. For physical healing, it is preferable to place your hands, if modestly possible, near the place of the problem, such as lower back, shoulder, neck or knee. It is also wise if the person doing the LOOH ministry is the same gender as the person receiving.

LOOH is normally accompanied by prayer. It can also be an occasion for a prophetic revelation and declaration.

Please, when you are asking for healing ministry, do not overload the praying person with a long description of all your problems and symptoms and negative history. All that will do is deplete their faith for your healing. It is better to simply say: "I am here to receive healing for my back (or whatever it is) from Jesus."

Similarly, when you are the minister who is going to pray the healing into being, get the recipient to focus on Jesus and the promises of God in His Word, not on their symptoms, problems or medical history.

Let my readers beware of and completely avoid and advise others against Reiki healing, which is the devil's counterfeit of the Lord's ministry.

> *"These signs will accompany those who have believed in My name .... they will lay hands on the sick, and they will recover."*
> *Mark 16:17–18*

I looked into the literal meaning of the Greek words that are translated as "recover". They actually mean that after the laying on of hands, the sick person will have and hold on to beauty, well-being, health, goodness, soundness, and rightness.

Remember we are the Body of Christ. When Jesus wants to stretch out His hands to heal, as He did Luke 4:40, He uses our hands.

When you do this, it will help you if you imagine Jesus' hands flowing through your hands. Imagine also the following picture from the prophet Habakkuk.

> [3] I see God moving ....
> [4] ... Rays of light flash from his hands, where his awesome power is hidden.
>
> *Habakkuk 3:3-4 NLT*

As you lay hands on someone for their healing, imagine this power being transferred to the sick person. If you are the sick one who is receiving ministry, imagine this divine power flowing into your body.

Examples of this ministry are: Matthew 8:3 &15; 9:29; Mark 6:5; 7:32-35; 9:27; Luke 4:40; 13:13; 22:51; Acts 3:7; 9:41; 28:8.

As God accelerates and perfects the process of recovery, it will be quicker than the body can do by itself and quicker than doctors expect.

The inclusion of this recovery process in the promises of God recognises that not all people are going to be completely healed the instant that they receive healing ministry.

The Lord is stretching their faith to bring their own healing to completion. God is teaching them to enforce Christ's victory by commanding the devil and the sickness to flee from them. Believers must learn to take authority over their own body by commanding the condition to be healed, the symptoms to stop and their body parts to be well and function normally, in Jesus' Name, Amen.

What is one thing you have learned from this teaching?

____

What is one thing you can do to implement this teaching?

____

Faith Declaration:

I thank You Lord that healing belongs to me because of Jesus. Thank You for providing a variety of means by which I can appropriate my healing. Right now I release my faith, for myself and for every believer who expresses their faith for healing through the means You have provided, to be free of every sickness, weakness and dysfunction, in Jesus' Name. Amen. Lord I lay hands on my own body and speak my healing into being in the Mighty Name of Jesus. I command my body to be well and every symptom of sickness, weakness and dysfunction to stop now and never return.

9 How God Heals part two

Testimony

In Atlanta, Georgia, USA a 62-year old lady with lots of needs stood for her healings. She had been getting neck and back treatment from chiropractors for many years. She had not been able to touch the floor for a long time. Her fingers were so swollen she could not wear her wedding and engagement rings. As she stepped out in faith to bend towards the floor, she was able to go so far down as to place her palms flat on the floor. She could move her neck freely any way she wanted without pain or restriction. She realised her fingers were more mobile, because some of them had been partly frozen. She also knew that some finger swelling had gone down. This faith-and-praise-filled woman of God was crying copious tears of joy. Hallelujah.

One thing about receiving healing remains the same: We must keep our faith in the Grace and Word of God. Miracles only happen by faith. (Galatians 3:5).

If God doesn't heal you one way, He will heal you another way.

In the previous chapter, I explained healing by the Word and by the Laying on of Hands.

(3) Calling the Elders to pray

The third method by which we can receive physical healing is by calling for the Elders of our local church to anoint us with oil and pray the prayer of faith for us.

> [14] *Is anyone among you sick? He must call for the elders (spiritual leaders) of the church and they are to pray over him, anointing him with oil in the name of the Lord;* [15] *and the prayer of faith will restore the one who is sick, and the Lord will raise him up; and if he has committed sins, he will be forgiven.*
>
> *James 5:14–15 AMPL*

You will notice the use of the word "must". This is important. It tells us that if we want to be healed we have to not only want that healing but also do something to get healed. One of the things we can do is to ask for the prayer of faith from other believers. In this case the sick person asks the Elders (recognized spiritual leaders) of his or her local church to minister to them.

The elders are asked to do two things: firstly, anoint the sick person with oil, which is usually done by placing some oil on the person's forehead, sometimes in the shape of the Cross; and secondly, pray the prayer of faith. If the elders do not have the faith to believe for your healing, then ask someone else to minister in this way to you.

(4) Anointing with Oil

Included in the previous method of healing is the ministry of Anointing with Oil. This method was used by the Twelve when Jesus sent them out.

> 7 *Calling the Twelve to him, he (Jesus) began to send them out two by two and gave them authority over impure spirits.*
> 12 *They went out and preached that people should repent.* 13 *They drove out many demons and anointed many sick people with oil and healed them.*
> *Mark 6:7,12–13*

Oil is a symbol of Holy Spirit. So using the oil is a prophetic act that says: "I believe Holy Spirit is going to quicken your mortal body for your healing as the result of this prayer of faith." (Romans 8:11).

(5) Confess to one another

This is linked to the need for us to have a healthy soul before we can receive our healing. (1 John 3:2).

It is also an acknowledgement of the fact that sin separates us from God and hinders our prayers. (Isaiah 59: 1–2; Psalm 66:18).

I can also tell you that sin lets the devil in. The devil brings sickness with him. King David experienced this and described his guilt, shame and sickness in Psalm 32:1–5.

The Epistle of James says:

> *14 Is anyone among you sick? ... 15 and if he has committed sins, they will be forgiven him. 16 Therefore, confess your sins to one another, and pray for one another so that you may be healed. The effective prayer of a righteous man can accomplish much.*
>
> *James 5:14–16 NASB*

Notice that the onus is on the sick person to put their faith into action, by confessing their sins, faults, mistakes, hurts, offences and other negatives and by asking for healing, believing that as they and the elders act upon the Word of God, the Lord will indeed heal the sick.

Again I say: When we do what the Bible says, God will do what the Bible says.

I want to point out something to you based upon the NIV translation:

> *"The prayer of a righteous man is powerful*
> *and effective.*
> *James 5:16 NIV.*

This verse, in its context, is about your and my effectiveness in healing ministry. You have been made righteous in Christ. So, your prayers are powerful and effective ! Hallelujah.

Another passage that links living righteously with healing is:

> 7 *..... Fear the LORD and turn away from evil.*
> 8 *It will be healing to your body*
> *and refreshment to your bones.*
>
> *Proverbs 3:7–8*

Different Bible versions translate the things we need to confess as sins, transgressions, faults and offences. In other words, getting rid of every negative thing inside you will assist you in receiving your healing, just as it did King David.

When we keep things hidden in secret, in the dark, we allow the devil to infect us with things like guilt, condemnation, depression, shame and fear. Our sin gives the devil the opportunity to afflict us. He can also keep us in spiritual, emotional and mental deception and bondage. This also allows him to lock us in a prison of bad attitudes, bad habits and sickness. Remember, Jesus treated all sickness as the work of the devil, not of God. (Acts 10:38).

When we bring things into the light, as we do with confession, God can then work His mighty works of righteousness, peace, freedom and healing. This is because He, and not the devil, is now Lord of the situation. Our newly healthy soul now contributes to us having a healthy body. This is the principle of James 5:15-16 and 1 John 3:2. Hallelujah.

(6) Communion

This most beautiful and powerful Christian experience of remembrance, thanksgiving, praise, love and faith is also a time of exchange. We exchange our life for His life, our sin for His righteousness, our foolishness for His wisdom, our weakness for His strength, our sickness for His healing, our mourning for His joy, our ashes for His beauty etc etc etc.

At Communion we recognize afresh Who Jesus is, what Jesus did for us, Who He is in us and who we are in Him.

Jesus Himself taught us that "Healing is the Children's Bread" in His encounter with the Syrophoenician mother who refused to let Him say "no" to the deliverance of her daughter. (Matthew 15:26). Of course, Jesus described Himself as the Bread of Life and He did so in language that echoes the Communion sacrament He was to later institute. (John 6:47–58).

Jesus also taught us to ask for our daily bread. (Matthew 6:11). That surely includes our healing, because we cannot live our daily life to the full, as God intends, without the bread of healing being a reality in our lives.

I have heard testimonies of people who experienced healing by taking the Communion emblems of bread and red grape juice daily in faith for that Divine exchange of His life of health replacing their life of sickness.

The classic Communion passage in 1 Corinthians 11:23–34 has much to teach us. Let's focus on 3 of those verses.

> 29 For anyone who eats and drinks [without solemn reverence and heartfelt gratitude for the sacrifice of Christ], eats and drinks a judgment on himself if he does not recognize the body [of Christ].
> 30 That [careless and unworthy participation] is the reason why many among you are weak and sick, and a number sleep [in death].
> 31 But if we evaluated and judged ourselves honestly [recognizing our shortcomings and correcting our behaviour], we would not be judged.
>
> *1 Corinthians 11:29–31 AMPL*

This is not an easy passage to understand. In the context, it seems to be dealing with the situation where many guests came to a Communion meal. The earlier guests ate their fill and were getting drunk on the wine. The later guests (in those times that would mean poorer invitees who were just getting home from work) missed out on getting a fair share of the meal and drink. The concept of equality (rather than rich versus poor) is significant, because it represents all being one in Christ. (Galatians 3:26–29).

It is a pretty tough judgement if the passage is interpreted in that light, because it would be saying the early and greedy (and probably proud and rich) guests could get weak, sick and even die.

Another way of looking at the passage is to say that those who contribute to disunity in the local church, the Body of Christ (1 Corinthians 11:18), are the unworthy ones who could get weak, sick and even die. I must say that, in my experience as a local church senior pastor during three decades of ministry, I have known a lot of people in various churches who contributed to division, but I cannot recall even one that was recognized as becoming weak, sick or dying because of their lack of unity or refusal to submit to godly leadership or their divisive, manipulative leadership style.

My preferred way of interpreting this passage hinges on my understanding of Communion in the context of the whole Bible.

The Passover in Exodus 12, tells us symbolically that the Blood of Jesus protects us from sickness and death. The testimony of the bronze snake in the wilderness teaches us that when we look to what Jesus did for us on the cross we will be saved and healed. (Numbers 21:4–9; John 3:14–15).

I therefore believe the expression "discerning the Lord's Body" (KJV and YLT. A footnote to the NLT says "other manuscripts read *the Lord's body.*") is talking about Jesus' literal physical body and what Jesus did for us (according to Isaiah 53:4–5). I do not consider that the primary meaning of this Communion passage is related to the church, the Body of Christ.

Therefore the meaning of 1 Corinthians 11:29–31 is this: if you do not recognise what Jesus did for you on the Cross, especially in regard to the forgiveness of your sins, the healing of your body and the transformation of your life as He comes to live in you (Galatians 2:20; 1 John 4:4), then you could be weak, sick and even die because you are not living a worthy, faith–filled, Christian – that is, Christ–centred – life.

It follows that if you live a worthy Christian lifestyle of love for and faith in Jesus, He will protect you as in the Passover and heal you as in the wilderness. Healing is indeed the Children's bread and when you as a child of God partake of the Communion bread in this worthy way, you will be healed. Amen.

What is one thing you have learned from this teaching?

____

What is one thing you can do to implement this teaching?

____

Faith Declaration:

I thank You Father for Your Grace and what Your Son has done for me. I am grateful for my inheritance in Christ, including my healing. I thank you for providing the means for me to receive my healing manifest in my body and for Your Indwelling Holy Spirit keeping me in good health. As I take Communion now, I confess my sins, I repent of my bad attitudes, I ask forgiveness for my resentments, unforgiveness and for times when I have hurt or offended others. I come to exchange my life, by faith for Christ's life, my sinfulness for His righteousness; my messes and mistakes for His miracles; my ashes for His beauty and prosperity; my mourning and depression for his joy; my over-sensitivity toward myself and under-sensitivity to others for His sensitivity both to God and people; my sickness for His healing; and my weakness for His strength, in Jesus' Name. Amen.

10 How God Heals part three

Testimony

At one meeting in Augusta, Georgia, USA, I had a word of knowledge about someone present with a neck problem. Holy Spirit showed me exactly where the pain was being felt. Pastor Gerry responded and was healed as I laid hands on his neck. He had been injured by being rear-ended when his pick-up truck was stationary.

A lady named Brandy was there who had been invited by the host Pastor. She was sitting in the second row from the front. She turned around to the back of the church to see what God was doing for Pastor Gerry. As she moved her neck, the Lord healed her of a neck problem she had endured for 12 years. Hallelujah.

(7) Special prayer.

The first of God's Ways of healing we will look at in this chapter is special prayer.

Our lifestyle of two-way prayer with the Lord includes praise and worship and waiting on God. This is not something the bulk of the Western church is noted for. Let us remember prayer is not something we have to do, it is something we are privileged to do. Two-way prayer between the Christian and the Lord is the means by which our faith syphons the Divine blessings, revelation, power and provision God's grace makes available to us, from heaven to earth. Special prayer is when we go beyond our normal "routine" of prayer and put some extra faith, focus, persistence and dedication into our pursuit of our desired answer.

- Hannah's answered prayer to conceive Samuel is an example of special intensity in prayer being rewarded. (1 Samuel 1:10-20). Times of focussed and soaking prayer, praise and worship are necessary in some instances. This will often be the case when a miracle is needed.

- Special persistence and faith in prayer is rewarded in the accounts of Jacob wrestling with God (Genesis 32: 24-30) and in the deliverance of the Syro-Phonecian mother's daughter. Jacob said: I will not let You go until You bless me. The mother simply would not take "no" for an answer from the Lord. (Matthew 15:22-28). She ignored His silence and His declaration of her lack of qualifications. She knew Jesus was her only answer. This mother teaches us to not lose faith when God is silent, nor when we are attacked by feelings of unworthiness. God is always for us. He always has good plans for us. We are declared worthy in Christ.

Jesus' parable of the woman and the unjust judge in Luke 18:1–8 teaches the same principle of God rewarding persistence in prayer. This does not mean religiously, mindlessly and meaninglessly repeating the same prayer over and over. Effective persistence in prayer is about fervently demanding your New Covenant rights, based on what Jesus did for you and on the promises and principles of God's Word.

- Special length of prayer is rewarded in Daniel 10:1–14, when the prophet prayed for 21 days. In Exodus 34:29–35 we read that Moses spent so much time in the Presence of God that his face shone with imparted and reflected glory. When we spend quality and quantity time with God, we are changed (2 Corinthians 3:18) and God imparts His revelation, blessing and resources to us. (Psalm 16:11).

- Special prayer partnership is rewarded in Exodus 17:8–15. This was when Moses, Aaron and Hur prayed together, thereby empowering Joshua to defeat the Amalekites in battle. The same principle and reward is passed on to New Covenant believers in Matthew 18:19–20.

(8) Special Prayer and Fasting

> *25 .. Jesus ... rebuked the unclean spirit, saying to it, "You spirit that won't let him talk or hear—I command you to come out of him and never enter him again!" 26 The*

> *spirit screamed, shook the child violently, and came out. ...[28] When Jesus came home, his disciples asked him privately, "Why couldn't we drive the spirit out?"[29] He told them, "This kind can come out only by prayer and fasting."*
> *Mark 9:25–29*

Fasting is one of the things Jesus said the Father would see us doing in private and would openly reward us for doing (Matthew 6: 18).

I have always believed it is significant that the first sin in the Garden of Eden involved the eating of forbidden food. That sin enabled the devil to usurp the delegated authority over the earth God had given to Adam. So, it is not a surprise to me that fasting facilitates us exercising authority over the devil, as Jesus did during His wilderness temptations. (Luke 4:1–14).

It is also important to note that Jesus' time of fasting and fighting the devil in the wilderness led to Him going from the fullness of the Spirit in Luke 4:1 to the power of the Spirit in Luke 4:14. Fasting helps us access the power and victory of God. But you should not think that fasting is designed to twist God's arm, as if he was reluctant to bless us or answer our prayers.

Fasting is a way of showing God that you are putting Him first in your life (Matthew 6:33) and that you are earnestly seeking Him. (Hebrews 11:6).

Please do not fast from food and forget to pray. Please do not fast from food and spend all day thinking about food instead of the Lord and His Word. You would be better off to fast from television, Facebook or video games and give that time to worship, waiting on the Lord, intercession and reading the Bible.

Jesus was emphasising a lifestyle of quality prayer, with fasting at times, as being the only way to evict such a strong demon. A lifestyle of two-way prayer is necessary for successful ministry. This is exemplified by the prophet Daniel and prophetess Anna in Luke 2:36–38.

Some people need more than one prayer to come through to complete healing. Some miracles require significant prayer and fasting before they become real in someone's earthly circumstances. The question is how much do you want that miracle, that breakthrough, that complete and permanent healing? Will you pray the price for the prize in a lifestyle way and through special prayer, as Paul said he did in Philippians 3:12–14.

Remember, too, that Paul said he spoke in tongues more than all the Corinthians. (1 Corinthians 14:18). This is perfect prayer, because Holy Spirit is speaking to God through you. This should be part of your lifestyle and special prayer. I believe this is one reason why Paul had one of the greatest healing and miracle ministries in the entire 2,000 year long (so far) church age. He was truly yielded to the control of Holy Spirit. Therefore, Holy Spirit had full and free access to bring Heaven to earth through the great apostle.

The other kind of prayer that is most likely to draw miracles from heaven to earth is praying the Scriptures back to God.

Too many people send the Lord junk prayers. They contain too much complaining and too long descriptions of their problems. God knows what you need before you ask Him. He knows how you got sick and why and what is needed for you to receive your healing.

How wonderful instead to pray like Jeremiah did in chapter 32 verse 17 (through to 25) of the book he penned. The Lord quoted Jeremiah's prayer back to him in verse 26. Hallelujah. That's the kind of prayer which gets answers from God.

> 17 'Ah Lord God! Behold, You have made the heavens and the earth by Your great power and by Your outstretched arm! Nothing is too difficult for You, ...
> 26 Then the word of the Lord came to Jeremiah, saying, 27 "Behold, I am the Lord, the God of all flesh; is anything too difficult for Me?"
> Jeremiah 32:17,26–27 NASB

I must say again that our asking God for healings and miracles is not just about repeating the same request time after time as if it was a ritual. (Matthew 6:7–8).

The Greek word that is translated as "ask" in Matthew 7:7–8 and Luke 11:9–10 is not a weak word. The best literal meaning of "aiteo" I can give you is based on research I did that included the teachings of Preceptaustin.org and Donald Mann.

Aiteo means to ask God for something, being respectful of the fact that He is Lord (not impudent, as if we were ordering God to do something) and confident in the knowledge that He is Your rich and generous, all-powerful, faithful Heavenly Father.

Aiteo describes asking with intensity, with earnestness, fervour and passion and with a sense of urgency. It embraces the concept of demanding something, because you know you have a right to receive your answer.

Your right to receive your healing answer is based on two things: firstly, you are asking according to God's Will, which is described in His Word. (1 John 5:14-15); secondly, you have a New Covenant relationship and partnership with God, through Jesus who fulfilled the conditions of the New Covenant. By so doing, Jesus paid the price for every healing, miracle, blessing or resource you will ever need to receive from God. All these things are freely given to us by Grace (Romans 8:32); but it takes faith to receive them.. These things give you confidence in your praying.

Christians are not afraid that God might say "no", because Jesus has said "yes". (2 Corinthians 1:20). When we "aiteo" the Lord, we are expecting, almost requiring, a positive answer. This is because what we are asking for is something which is already ours by New Covenant promise. Jesus has already met all God's covenant requirements. Our prayers are answered because of Jesus performance. Our healing answers are not based on our performance, but they do require our faith.

Because of these meanings of "aiteo", when I pray, I often use that Greek word rather than the English word "ask", both in my spoken and written prayers.

(9) Gifts of Holy Spirit

> *[7] But to each one is given the manifestation of the Spirit [the spiritual illumination and the enabling of the Holy Spirit] for the common good. [8] To one is given through the [Holy] Spirit [the power to speak] the message of wisdom, and to another [the power to express] the word of knowledge and understanding according to the same Spirit; [9] to another [wonder-working] faith [is given] by the same [Holy] Spirit, and to another the [extraordinary] gifts of healings by the one Spirit; [10] and to another the working of miracles, and to another prophecy [foretelling the future, speaking a new message from God to the people], and to another discernment of spirits [the ability to distinguish sound, godly doctrine from the deceptive doctrine of man-made religions and cults], to another various kinds of [unknown]*

tongues, and to another interpretation of tongues. 11 All these things [the gifts, the achievements, the abilities, the empowering] are brought about by one and the same [Holy] Spirit, distributing to each one individually just as He chooses.
1 Corinthians 12:7-11 AMPL

Many people get healed through the operation of the spiritual gifts of Holy Spirit. As I explain in my book *"You Can Prophesy"*, these spiritual gifts can be used by any Christian who earnestly desires them. (1 Corinthians 14:1).

When I was first born again, I was not Spirit-filled, with the evidence of speaking in tongues. So I sought that experience. Then I pursued the prophetic gifts, which were imparted to me by the laying on of hands, after I got a rhema-word from God about that through Romans 1:11.

The next stage of my spiritual gifts development was to build upon my prophetic experience, because every gift is given to us in seed form. It's up to each believer to grow their gifts, just as in the parable of the talents. As I grew in Christ and in the Word of God, my ministry grew. By the Grace of God and faith, I am able to prophesy at a far greater level of accurate revelation than when I first began to prophesy.

My next step was to access the spiritual gift of the Word of Knowledge. That gift is important in both prophetic and healing ministry. Then I focused on having more Divine power in my life. I particularly pursued in prayer and ministry the spiritual gift of healing pain and all its causes.

The result has been many healings around Australia and internationally. People have been healed of conditions they have had for 40 years, 25 years, 8 years, 6 years etc.

These gifts are available to you both to receive your healing and to impart healing to others. They must be "earnestly desired". (1 Corinthians 12:31 and 14:1). Lukewarmness will never be enough to receive God's best. (Revelation 3:15-16 AMPL). So, aggressively seek the giftings of God for yourself. (Matthew 11:12). The Lord is even more desirous of blessing, healing and equipping than you will ever be to receive them. As long as you have the faith to receive, He has even greater grace to give.

(10) Gifted Ministers

We know healing is a ministry for every believer. However, there is no doubt that some, such as Reinhard Bonnke, Benny Hinn and Randy Clark are especially gifted in the ministry of healing, as were the apostles Paul and Peter in their day.

Going to the meetings and training events of gifted ministers could increase your faith to receive both healing and impartation of spiritual gifts.

Some ministers are especially gifted in certain, specific healings. I understand that the late C.P. Wagner had great success with skeletal needs and that Frank Houston was used by God to set many arthritis sufferers free.

As mentioned above, I sought the Lord for many years for the spiritual gift of healing pain and all its causes. One of the Scriptures that gave me faith was Isaiah 53:4 in which the Hebrew word "makob" specifically teaches that Jesus is our healer of pain problems. When I prayed I never asked simply for the healing of pain, but for the healing of the cause of the person's pain. Jesus is not Jehovah-Panadol or Jehovah-Advil or Jehovah-Tylenol. He does not just mask the pain and leave the condition unhealed. He is Jehovah Rapha, the Lord Who heals us. So when the pain goes, it is because you have been healed. Hallelujah.

As I have stepped out in faith time and time again, the Lord has given me great success in Australia and internationally in this ministry. However, I am hungry for the "much more" of God and the greater works of Jesus. (Matthew 7:11; Luke 11:13; John 14:12).

(11) Signs following the Preaching of the Word

This is true of every believer's ministry of the Word, especially in an evangelistic situation, whether we share the Gospel with one person or thousands. God turns up to show His power and glory and authority whenever and wherever there is a clash of kingdoms, between His Kingdom of Light and the devil's kingdom of darkness.

The revival in Samaria, inspired by the ministry of Philip the deacon-turned-evangelist, is a great example of this. (Acts 8:5-13).

(12) Through the Special Presence of the Lord

> One day Jesus was teaching, and Pharisees
> and teachers of the law were sitting there.
> They had come from every village of
> Galilee and from Judea and Jerusalem. And
> the power of the Lord was with Jesus to
> heal the sick.
> Luke 5:17

There are some Christian meetings when either the minister discerns a special anointing on him or her to heal the sick or many are aware of a powerful corporate anointing in the room. Faith is heightened and many are able to receive their healing.

This was certainly the case on many occasions in the great Asuza Street revival in Los Angeles at the turn of the 20th century. People were healed of deafness, blindness and there were even miracles of severed fingers that grew back to normal size and function.

(13) Prayer Cloths

> [11] *God was extraordinary miracles by the hands of Paul,* [12] so that handkerchiefs or aprons were even carried from his body to the sick, and the diseases left them and *the evil spirits went out.*
>
> *Acts 19:11–12*

This is a ministry that continues to the present day. There are many testimonies of ministers and local churches who have prayed over and sometimes anointed such cloths with oil. When the person takes them back to be placed upon sick people in homes and hospitals, healings have resulted.

(14) Through Medical and Natural means

It is notable that God has creatively included in human DNA the striving for restoration of health. This is a further indicator of the fact that healing is always the Will of God.

I believe that, as many tribal societies have proven, God put healing properties in various plants, again showing that He wants people healed. This is also a validation of medical treatments. It is also a fulfilment of the following Proverb.

> *It is the glory of God to conceal a matter, but the glory of kings is to search out a matter.*
> *Proverbs 25:2 NASB*

I have written more about medical healing in Chapter 16.

Scriptural examples include King Hezekiah's healing in Isaiah 38:21 and the advice Paul gave Timothy regarding the medicinal use of wine in
1 Timothy 5:23. Some might consider that part of Elisha's resurrection of the Shunammite woman's son included what we today call C.P.R. or cardiopulmonary resuscitation. (2 Kings 4:32–35).

King Asa's testimony teaches us to pray and not only rely on doctors and their treatments.

> 12 *In the thirty-ninth year of his reign Asa was afflicted with a disease in his feet. Though his disease was severe, even in his illness he did not seek help from the Lord,* but only from the physicians.
> 13 *Then in the forty-first year of his reign Asa died and rested with his ancestors.*
>
> *2 Chronicles 16:12–13*

Conclusion

These three chapters are included to say that just as Jesus healed people in different ways, so God has provided a variety of means whereby His people may experience Divine healing. It is up to us to pursue our healing by whatever means He has provided until it is effected in our bodies.

I must mention here the absolute importance of your earnest, active, persistent desire to be healed and faith for your healing. It is possible, as Peter demonstrated when walking on the water, to stop a miracle from manifesting fully, before it is complete. (Matthew 14:28–31).

So, please do not give up hope for, nor pursuit of your complete and permanent healing, because that is what Jesus paid for and won on your behalf.

Don't settle for some improvement. Keep actively believing for God's fullness.

Don't let the devil trick you with lies that are not according to the New Covenant Grace that is promised to you in the Word of God and that rob you of your healing. Don't yield to demonically initiated lying symptoms that come back after you have been healed. Submit to God; resist the devil and he will flee from you. (James 4:7).

Always trust the Nature and power of God to fulfil His Word in your life. Of course, this includes believing what the Bible teaches and promises. Jeremiah 1:12 says that

God is "watching over My word to perform it." (see also Isaiah 55:11; Psalm 107:20).

What is one thing you have learned from this teaching?

What is one thing you can do to implement this teaching?

Faith Declaration:

I thank You Lord for the fact that You are a prayer-answering, miracle-working God. I praise You for Your goodness and greatness. I give you glory because You are so eager to bless, transform and equip Your people. I thank You because You give Your healing unconditionally by Grace, because of Jesus. Praise Him. By faith I receive my healing now. I command my body to be well now and in good health for the rest of my life, in Jesus' Name. Amen. I also ask for the gifts of Holy Spirit to heal others that You may be glorified and many people healed to testify that Jesus Christ is Lord. I declare in faith that as I pray for others, and lay hands on them, You will heal them for Jesus' sake. Amen.

11 How to receive your Healing part one

Testimony

Paul came to the meeting in Orlando, Florida, USA. He had pain in his neck and lower back from a degenerated disc and a pinched nerve. He also had some chest pains. He felt the Lord touch him as he sat in the congregation and he also came to the front of the church for ministry. He said that as I prayed for him all his pain left him. He testified to another member of the congregation that he was "free" and confessed that his healing was "permanent" in Jesus' Name.

The first thing you must do to receive your healing is to build your faith in the specific area of believing for your body to be healed.

> *Only Faith can guarantee the blessings we hope for or prove the existence of realities that at present remain unseen*
>
> *Hebrews 11:1 Jerusalem Bible*

> *What is Faith? It is the confident assurance that something we want is going to happen. It is the certainty that what we hope for is waiting for us even though we cannot see it up ahead.*
>
> *Hebrews 11:1 Living Bible*

Let me define some characteristics of faith for you with this acronym.

FAITH IS

- Founded on God and His Nature.
- He is the all-powerful, always-good and grace-giving Lord Who provides for your every need and righteous-desire, including your healing. Our faith makes possible all that God is capable of. The Bible teaches that there is nothing too big or too small for God and no-one is out of His reach.

- Active confidence in God's Word.

This means living by and acting in faith. (Romans 1:17; James 2:17)

Faith is knowing the Will of God and doing it. Faith is hearing the Voice of God and obeying it.

Faith can be described as confidence in God. (Hebrews 10:35). One of the ways this manifests is by the believer having the strong expectation that God will show up when we step out in faith. The expression Holy Spirit gave me that encapsulates this concept is: "When you do what the Bible says, God will do what the Bible says."

A plaque on my desk says: "Faith is not believing God can, it is knowing that He will."

Continuing and growing faith is based on you continuing and growing in the Word of God. (John 8:31 NASB).

- In Love with and In touch with the Lord.

Faith is all about our relationship and partnership with God. We are King's kids, His adopted sons and daughters.

We have the Lord's favour. We have access to Him and to all that is His. We have the benefits of sonship, not only in terms of inheritance, but also delegated authority.

In Christ, we are empowered to do the works of God on earth and by so doing to bring the Kingdom and the blessings, resources and conditions of heaven to earth.

In terms of healing, as a son or daughter of God you have the right to be healed and to minister healing, even to yourself.

- Total Trust, as a child of your perfect Heavenly Father.

You know God will never hurt you, leave you, fail you or forget you.

We trust God not only in good times, but also when we are in situations that we do not want, nor understand.

> *Trust in and rely confidently on*
> *the LORD with all your heart*
> *And do not rely on your own*
> *insight or understanding.*
> *6 In all your ways know and*
> *acknowledge and recognize Him,*
> *And He will make your paths*
> *straight and smooth [removing obstacles*
> *that block your way].*
>
> *Proverbs 3:5-6 AMPL*

There are times when you all you can do is "be still and know" that He is God (Ps. 46:10a), because there seems to be nothing you can do to make your prayer come true. This is the time we are really tested on whether we will walk by faith, not by sight (2 Corinthians 5:7), nor by feelings.

- Holding on to God and His Word, no matter what, or how long it takes for your miracle to become a reality in our material world.

We do not want you to become lazy, but to imitate those who through faith and patience inherit what has been promised.

Hebrews 6:12 NIV

so that you will not be [spiritually] sluggish, but [will instead be] imitators of those who through faith [lean on God with absolute trust and confidence in Him and in His power] and by patient endurance [even when suffering] are [now] inheriting the promises.

Hebrews 6:12 AMPL

Please understand that patience is not hanging around doing nothing. Patience is enduring in well-doing, while you are waiting for the manifestation of your blessing.

According to Mark 11:24, you need to believe that what you have asked for is already yours; in other words, it is already real and credited to your account in the spiritual world of the Kingdom of God. Sometime after you have reached that point of faith, it will become manifest. One of the ways, you exercise faith in this regard is to stop asking God for it and begin to thank Him for it. Abraham grew to full assurance of faith by giving glory to God before he was healed and before Isaac was conceived and born. (Romans 4:19-21).

There has been much teaching over the years about the difference between the LOGOS-word of God, which is the written Bible and the RHEMA-word of God, which is the specific word from the Word that inspires your faith (according to Romans 10:17). The RHEMA-word may be a specific revelation from the Father (Matthew 4:4) or from Holy Spirit (according to Ephesians 6:17b) that becomes your sword of the Spirit, which enables you to enforce Christ's victory over the problem/s you are facing.

In a similar way, we must have faith that is specific to the need we have, rather than just general faith. Sometimes people think they did have faith for something but it still didn't happen.

I heard a preacher named Mac Hammond once give these four indicators of a faith that is not yet ready to receive the miracle that is being believed for. This is an adapted explanation of his four points.

(1) Fear is just as present in the person as faith. Doubt and fear are great hindrances to faith;

(2) The person will not (although they might say: "I can not") believe unless and until they first see it or feel it. Remember we are to walk and receive our healings and other miracles by faith, not by sight, nor by feelings. (2 Corinthians 5:7). The very definition of faith in Hebrews 11:1 tells us that faith is the evidence of things not seen.

(3) The person is doubtful of God meeting their need in the NOW of their experience. Again I say: Doubt and fear are great hindrances to faith.

(4) The person's mouth is not full of Bible-fuelled, New Covenant-based, Christ-centred faith and only

faith. In Luke 6:45, Jesus taught that the heart is what fills our mouths. In other words, what we say is an indication of what is in our heart, what is deep within, what we truly believe. If you do not have faith within, your words will not be words of faith. If you do not have faith within, you are not ready to receive your healing or other miracle.

How to grow your Faith for Healing

(1) According to Romans 10:17, faith comes from hearing the Word of God. So read the Bible, especially the Gospels and the Book of Acts, regularly.

(2) As you read God's Word, ask Holy Spirit to renew your mind about Divine healing. Reject doubt, fear and unbelief that are fuelled by the devil, by the sophisticated, educated cynicism of this world, by the unbelief of people in your sphere of influence and by the disappointment of things that did not work out as you wanted them or are taking a long time to come to pass.

(3) Buy teaching series on healing or watch them on YouTube.

(4) Learn the key verses in the Bible that promise healing. Speak those verses out loud. Put your name in them.

(5) Visualise yourself in the healing miracles of the Bible, both receiving and giving healing.

(6) Imagine Christ in you reaching out through your words and hands and faith and love to heal people you

are ministering to. Imagine people saying "I am healed; I am healed" after you have ministered to them in Jesus' Name.

(7) Answers to prayer build your faith, so be a doer of the Word and pray for the sick. Their healing testimonies will grow your faith. The Lord taught me this principle which I often get congregations to repeat after me. I encourage you to say this out loud now, as you are reading this page:

"When I do what the Bible says, God will do what the Bible says."

That principle and faith confession will help you both receive healing and minister healing to others.

(8) Go to God for His Divine impartation of the faith of God. (Mark 11:22 Young's Literal Translation. See also Aramaic Bible in Plain English and Berean Literal Bible). Ask the Lord for the spiritual gifts of Holy Spirit, including faith and healing. (1 Corinthians 12:9).

(9) Attend healing conferences and receive impartation through the Lord's anointed servants.

(10) Receive the training for and then join a prayer ministry team in your local church or in an interdenominational healing ministry in your locality.

(11) Pray, praise and thank the Lord for His healing ministry, His power and His grace.

(12) Build the Holy Spirit fruit of faith and faithfulness in your life as you live by faith, in obedience to God's

Word, as a lifestyle. The Greek word *"pistis"* in Galatians 5:22 is normally translated as "faith" in that verse, but many Bible versions substitute "faithfulness" for "faith". Both are the fruit of the Spirit. As you grow in God over the long haul, you will grow in both faith and faithfulness.

(13) Keep focussing on who you are in Christ according to the Word of God and Who Christ is in you.

(14) To emphasise what I said in point (4), keep speaking out loud as declarations of your faith that release Holy Spirit into action, all the healing verses you find in the Scriptures. Remember to put your name in them. Command your body to come into line with these promises of God.

What is one thing you have learned from this teaching?

____

What is one thing you can do to implement this teaching?

____

Faith Declaration:

I praise You Lord for Your perfect character and infinite power and authority. I honour You for Your Covenant-keeping commitment to Your word and Your people. I thank You that You say what You mean and mean what You say and do what You say. I praise You that Jesus has said "yes" to every promise in Your Word. I now say the "amen" to my healing because by Jesus' wounds I am healed. I am grateful that healing belongs to me because Jesus purchased it for me by His suffering and triumph. I declare by faith that it is finished; my healing is done. By faith I draw out of the spiritual realm what is mine into the reality of my physical body. I command my body to be well and every symptom of sickness, weakness and dysfunction to cease now and never return. I declare the devil is a defeated foe and I command his thieving and destruction to stop now and full restoration to be mine, because Jesus came to give me abundant life. Hallelujah.

12 How to receive your healing part two

Testimony

Mikka's shoulder had dislocated six times. It was painful on a daily basis. She was waiting for surgery. It was restricting her work performance. After the healing ministry time, she demonstrated the fact that she was pain free, had completely unrestricted movement. Mikka could not only move her shoulder and arm in a full range of directions but she showed that she could put further pressure on it, stretching it beyond its normal limits, without any pain or problem. She was so very happy and it showed. Mikka gave the Lord glory for what He had done for her, which she was able to receive that Sunday morning in Glossop, in the Riverland area of South Australia.

In the last chapter I emphasised that you must build and focus your faith specifically on receiving your Divine healing. There are three very important keys to doing this.

3 Keys to releasing your Faith for Healing

The first key is realising Jesus has already done all He needed to do for you to be healed. When He said on the Cross "It is Finished", one of the things that was included in that statement was your healing. When you get sick, Jesus does not have to be lashed again or climb back on to the Cross. What He had to do for you to be healed He has done.

The second key is found in the fact that if you had been alive 2,000 years ago and had been present any one of the twelve times Jesus unconditionally healed everyone who was where He was, you too would have been immediately, completely and permanently healed. The Good News is that you don't have to go back in time for that to happen, because He has come forward to our time.

> *8 Jesus Christ is [eternally changeless, always] the same yesterday and today and forever.*
> *Hebrews 13:8 AMPL*

The third key is that where you are, He is.

> *For where two or three have gathered together in My name, I am there in their midst."*
>
> *Matthew 18:20 NASB*

When I am ministering healing to a congregation, I will often quote this Scripture and ask the people if they believe it. Of course, the Christians present all say: "Yes, we believe it." Then I say: "I am not sure I believe you."

I say that because, if we really believed Jesus is in the room with us, then we should have the faith to receive healing from Him, just as everyone did 2,000 years ago. The difference is that they could see Him with their natural eyes, but we can't. We are in the situation Jesus described to the apostle Thomas.

> *Jesus said, "So, you believe because you've seen with your own eyes. Even better blessings are in store for those who believe without seeing."*
> *John 20:29 MSG*

The thing is, that just believing Jesus is in the room with you is not enough. You must by faith draw His power from Him to meet your need. Blind Bartimaeus shouted to get Jesus' attention and received his healing as his reward. (Mark 10:46–52). However, when Jesus healed the lame man at the Pool of Bethesda, there is no record of other needy people crying out "Lord, heal me." The testimony of the Gospels is that if any of the others in the vicinity of the Pool had called out for healing while Jesus was there, Jesus would have healed them.

So you must aggressively (which does not mean loudly) pursue your healing when you believe Jesus is in the room with you. Remember that God is the great "I AM", the God of the "now".

There were occasions when Jesus acted as if He would bypass the disciples unless they called upon Him. (Mark 6:48–51; Luke 24:28–29). So, you and your faith must connect with the Lord when the moment and opportunity for healing is upon you. That's what the woman with the issue of blood did. She received her healing, not just because she physically touched Jesus, as so many others did that day, but because she touched the Lord by her faith. (Luke 8:43–48).

This leads me to another thing you can do to receive your healing. Just as that woman set herself a "point of contact" for her faith, so can you. I remember reading a book of miracle testimonies by Benny Hinn. In a number of those amazing healings the sick person said: If I go to this meeting, I will be healed." And they were. They believed before they went, while they were there, during the praise and worship, the announcements, the offering, the preaching and the ministry time. They believed before they received, when they received and after they received.

I want to also comment on something the angel said to Cornelius.

> *The angel answered, "Your prayers and gifts to the poor have come up as a memorial offering before God.*
>
> *Acts 10:4*

I am not a believer in the "prosperity Gospel". I do believe God provides for us and that He does so in a way which gives us the opportunity to bless others. (2 Corinthians 9:6–8). Maybe all we can share is a little flour and oil. (1 Kings 17:8–16). Perhaps we donate to foreign missions projects, such as church planting, orphanages and well-digging. Of course, the first and normal thing we do is to bring our whole tithes (10%) into the storehouse of our local church, where we are taught the Word of God and cared for by shepherds of integrity.

My point is this: I am a believer in the Law of Sowing and Reaping. God will reward our lifestyle of love, faith and obedience to His Word. Just as Cornelius was rewarded with his miracle, so the Lord will also reward you with yours. (Hebrews 11:6).

Word-based Imagination will help you release your Faith for Healing

There is a fourth matter I want to share with you, before I focus on receiving your healing. Some people may consider it to be controversial. It is the use of your imagination. It should not be controversial because imagination is part of our human creativity; it is a gift, an ability, from God. Imagination is a quality that of all living things only man has. It is part of our God-like-ness. (Genesis 1:26-27). God used His imagination to pre-plan all creation, the galaxies of stars and planets, His angelic host, the living things and creatures on earth (the biota, flora and fauna), the mountains, rivers, deserts, clouds etc etc. Then He spoke it all into existence.

When God imagined humans, He decided what aspects of His own Divine Nature He would include in man, such as the ***unlimited*** ability to choose (Note: I do not believe He gave that quality to the angels). God also pre-planned those qualities He would not impart to us, such as His Own Omnipotence or Omniscience or flight.

God did give us a spirit (because He is Spirit), a soul (mind, will, emotions), a body, a conscience and the ability to imagine and to envision things so that we could become creators as He is – but we cannot create things "ex nihilo" from nothing as He can and did.

Too many people only use imagination in childhood as an exercise of the soul. They fail to recognise it can be used in adulthood in the spirit realm.

> *Faith is the confidence that what we hope for will actually happen; it gives us assurance about things we cannot see.*
> *Hebrews 11:1 NLT*

Hope is seeing with our inner being what we cannot see with our physical eyes. There are two inner faculties that enable us to see what cannot be seen physically. They are our spirit, which is ignited prophetically by Holy Spirit; and our imagination, which bridges the soul and spirit. In regard to receiving your healing, it is initiated by visualising the Word of God being manifest in your life.

You see yourself in one of the healing passages in the Gospels. You imagine going to your Lord and Divine physician, Jesus. You imagine Him touching whatever part of your body needs healing. You imagine Divine power flowing out of Jesus into your body, restoring you to complete health and strength. Imagine your body part being healed. By faith you receive that healing and say: "Thank You Lord for healing me today. Amen."

Faith springs out of the soil of hope. If you can hope for something, then you can believe for it to become a reality in your life. Elisha asked for a double portion of Elijah's anointing. He had to see it, in order to receive it.

Hope gives us eyes to see the invisible, to see what is not yet a reality in our "now". Hope springs from what we see in the Word of God. Hope imagines what we see in the Word as a "not-yet" reality in our lives. Hope sees us healthy, with no physical ailments or impediments. Hope sees us walking, carrying, living pain-free. Then our faith says: "Amen to that."

When we truly believe that what we see by hope-fuelled imagination, based on the promises of God in His Word, is truly our inheritance in Christ, then our miracle will surely manifest. Faith makes real what hope sees.

So, when the time for healing ministry comes, it may help you to visualise Jesus as the One Who is touching you by the laying on of hands. After all, He is inside the Christian who is doing so, even when you lay hands on yourself. We Christians are Jesus' hands in this world.

Three Conditions I ask People to Implement

There are three conditions I always ask of the congregation before I minister healing to them.

(1) Stand for healing, not for prayer. If you stand or come forward for prayer, you will receive a prayer and sit back down with your answer, which is a prayer, not a healing. It is unlikely that you will receive your healing, because that is not what you asked for.

(2) Stand in Faith, not in Hope. Hope defers your healing to some other future time. It's as if you are thinking: "Lord You might be too busy or exhausted to get to my need now. But I am believing that one day, when You are not on holidays, nor on strike, nor too tired, nor too busy that I will get to the top of your "to-do" list. Then, if I am still in Your good books, and You are in a good mood, You will heal me on the unknown future day." You can understand without me needing to

comment further on this, that wishing and hoping with attitudes like these won't get you healed.

The name of the Lord that was revealed to Moses ("I AM" in Exodus 3:14) is important to our understanding of the fact that faith is "Now", whereas hope is future. You must stand for healing now. You must believe that Jesus will heal you right here, right now.

The Name "I AM" has three important meanings. Firstly, it tells us that God is the I AM, the Only UN-created Being in the universe and throughout eternity past, present and future.

Secondly, it signifies the Lord's absolute and infinite power and His unlimited generosity. In other words, God is saying to us through His name "I AM" that He is the Provider of anything and everything we will ever need. Think of it this way: I AM .... (Fill in the blank with whatever you need). For example: I AM your Healer; I AM your Peace; I AM your Victory; I AM your Counsellor/Teacher/Guide; I AM your Strength; I AM your financial Provider etc etc

Thirdly, the Name "I AM" clearly says: I AM your God, Who is in the Now of your needs and experience.

So, we need to connect our faith with God for our healing NOW, not at some later, future date.

I want to emphasise here that standing in faith now, and not in hope for a future healing is a key aspect of receiving the healing Jesus has already paid for you to have.

I suggest that you release your faith by imagining that Jesus is indeed in the room right now, with you and for you, just as Matthew 18:20 says.

Jesus is our Emmanuel, God with us. When we are together with Him in united faith, no prayer request will go unanswered. (Matthew 18:19).

So, in order to get healed, you choose to believe that Jesus is there for you to be healed, just as He was in the many Bible accounts where He healed everyone who came to Him of everything they had wrong with them. Jesus did this absolutely and unconditionally, not on the basis of each person's "naughty or nice" or "religious" behaviour.

It is impossible for us to go back and be in the room or field with Jesus when he healed "all" (Note: there are 17 records of this in the Gospels). The Good News is that we don't have to go back in time to get healed, because Jesus has come forward to our time. Jesus is alive and "the same yesterday, today and forever". (Hebrews 13:8).

The important thing is that you must connect to the Lord Who is in the room, not the preacher or prophet or healing minister. You must touch Jesus by faith as the woman with the issue of blood did. (Matthew 9:20). Others touched Jesus that day but not by faith, so they did not get healed when she did. On another occasion, people must have heard her testimony and in sincere faith copied her action of touching the hem of His garment, because they got healed too. (Matthew 14:36).

When Jesus was walking on the road to Emmaus, Jesus acted as if He would keep going. Like Blind Bartimaeus, His two companions had to persuade the Lord, to come in to the inn with them, where He continued to minister to them. (Luke 24:28–31). You need to make personal, individual contact with Jesus by faith when He is in the room with you, in order to receive your full healing.

(3) Try to do what you could not do before. In Matthew 12:13, Jesus told the man with the withered arm to do something he could not do, namely, "Stretch out your hand." The man could have said: "I can't." If he had, he would not have been healed. You might say: "it will hurt too much." Then, you won't get healed.

Movements like these are faith actions, by which you move against your problem and move into your miracle healing, as the man with the withered arm did. "The man reached out and it was restored, as normal *and* healthy ..." (Matthew 12:13 AMPL).

I have said to people and I say to you, **don't over-do this faith step**. For example, bend your back slowly and gently. Don't try to touch your toes in one quick movement and simultaneously pick up the nearest heavy weight you find.

I have previously written about the awesome, Divine power that is released by the words of our mouth. In Genesis chapter 1, Holy Spirit hovered over the earth creating an atmosphere of Divine power and authority, such as we experience in worship. When God spoke, Holy Spirit moved from atmosphere to action. When the Word of God is preached and when you speak the Word of God to your own body, Holy Spirit moves from atmosphere to action in your life.

In my book "*34 Faith-Lifters that Bless and Build Believers*" I wrote two chapters on this subject. The key verses you should look up are: Proverbs 12:14; 18:20-21; Job 22:21,26-28; Ezekiel 37:1-10.

How do you release this Divine power and cause Holy Spirit to spring into action? By simultaneously, as you do whatever physical faith steps are relevant to your healing, verbally thanking the Lord for your healing and commanding your body to be completely and permanently free of every pain and symptom and to function normally for the rest of your life, in Jesus' Name. Amen.

What is one thing you have learned from this teaching?

___

What is one thing you can do to implement this teaching?

___

Faith Declaration:

I praise You Lord Jesus for Your work on and after the Cross. You said: "it is finished." I believe Your suffering and triumph has purchased my healing for me. I thank You that healing belongs to me, because of You and the Grace of God. Lord I declare that according to Your Word, You are here with me and for me. By faith I see Your hand on my life and Your power flowing into my body. I receive my healing by faith and command my body to be well and stay well, with no symptoms of sickness, weakness or dysfunction, in Jesus' Name. Amen.

13 How to receive your healing part three

Testimony

In Derry (aka Londonderry), Northern Ireland, Damien came forward for the laying on of hands after receiving a touch from God in the congregation. He was healed of back pain, pins and needles in both his legs and pain in his left leg. A week later, the Pastor emailed me: "A 16-year-old girl in church that night had severe pain in her chest for 18 months. This restricted her ability to do many things. She testified several days later that she is pain-free and can now do the exercise she was previously unable to do."

- Be God-conscious, not self-conscious, nor focused on your symptoms.

- Be confident that healing belongs to you because of Jesus.
- Focus on Who Jesus is, what He did for you and that He is in the room with you and for you.
- As you visualise receiving your touch from the Lord, begin thanking God for your healing.
- Confess the Word of God with your mouth, for example: "By Your wounds, Lord, I am healed." Isaiah 53:5
- Begin to move your body, where it has been hurting or restricted, as an act of faith, believing that you are healed.
- As you do this, command your body to be well, pain-free and fully flexible and strong, in Jesus' Name.

If you receive only a partial healing

When a person receives a partial healing, you can be sure of this: The Lord is *stretching* their faith!

The fact is that as much as I pray for complete, instant, permanent healings to occur, neither I nor anyone else can remove Mark 16:18b from the Bible. That verse talks about sick people recovering. The literal translation of the Greek "echo-kalos" – to recover, means to have and to hold on to health, well-being, goodness, soundness, rightness and beauty.

Let me point out here that you must believe what God heals stays healed. Abraham is a Biblical proof of this. After the healing of his own and Sarah's bodies, which enabled them to have their son Isaac, Abraham later had more children with his wife Keturah. (Genesis 25:1–2). Apart from when Jesus prayed a second time for a blind man, who at first received only a partial healing, there is no record in Jesus' ministry of someone coming back after their healing to be healed again. However, Jesus did issue the warning "stop sinning or something worse may happen to you." If you give the devil an opportunity to rob you of your healing or to put the sickness back on you, he will do it.

The bottom line in regard to Mark 16:18b is that there are always going to be some people who receive a partial healing during the ministry time. However, what they must do is remember that Jesus said: "It is finished." Jesus does not have to get whipped again, nor go back on the Cross in order for anyone to receive their full and complete healing.

I use the following illustration to help people understand that their full healing was paid for by Jesus but they must actively receive it: When Jesus taught us that everyone who asks, receives, He used a strong military word, "lambano", which is translated into English by the word "receives". (Matthew 7:8). It actually means to seize. Lambano is a very pro-active word, not a passive one. It is a word that means the person has to do something active by faith in order to receive what they have asked for.

Jesus taught the same principle in John 7:37–39. Jesus said if we are thirsty (for our blessing, our answer to prayer, our healing, our experience of Holy Spirit), we have to (actively) come to Him and drink by faith.

Imagine Jesus going to your local pizza shop and paying for a free pizza for everyone in your church or town. If somebody doesn't believe it, they won't go to receive it. If they think the pizza shop will deliver it without them claiming it, they will go hungry.

Maybe another person feels they are only worthy of a few slices or they think others are more deserving because there might be only a limited supply. They might think: "I am only going to get the pizza a bit at a time, some now, some at another time, some more after that."

The reality is that our healing (and any and every other blessing we need from the Lord) is completely paid for and fully available for us to seize by faith.

If your physical body only registers a partial improvement, you must by faith receive and seize your complete and permanent healing. Keep thanking the Lord for it and commanding your body to manifest it until it is a reality.

Even if it takes time for your body to be totally healed, stay motivated, stay in faith. Your persistence will overcome all devilish resistance.

In Ephesians 1:13–14 the Bible says Holy Spirit is our "deposit guaranteeing our inheritance". Translating this promise into the realm of healing means that when you get a little improvement in your body, this is the deposit that guarantees God wants you to receive, to seize, your complete, permanent healing.

A significant factor in Divine healing is: How much do you want it? If you really want God to do it, keep pursuing it. Use every means of healing that He has provided, until you have fully possessed your promised inheritance in Christ, just as Joshua and Israel possessed theirs centuries ago.

You must be convinced by the Word of God, especially from the Christ-centred perspective of the New Covenant expressed in Jesus' ministry in the Gospels, that God sent His Son so that all who believe can be made whole, in spirit, soul and body. Putting it simply, as Andrew Wommack has said: "God wants you well."

When Jesus came, He changed the way God deals with people. Under the Old Covenant God did put sickness on the disobedient and He initiated their defeat and impoverishment. Under the New Covenant of Grace, God does not do any of those things. Instead of using the stick, He uses the carrot and the honey to get stubborn mules like us to love and follow and obey Him and to build their faith to receive the unlimited blessings Jesus' priceless sacrifice and complete and permanent triumph purchased for us.

Assuming you are a true born-again Christian, when it comes to your healing, peace, blessing and resourcing in every area of life, Jesus has said YES to every promise in the Bible. (2 Corinthians 1:20). He also famously said on the Cross just before He yielded His Spirit to the Father "It is Finished", which meant many things, including the fact that your complete and permanent healing is fully paid for.

So, believe it; receive it by faith. Then act in faith by speaking it into being, by commanding your body to be well and by testing your body out, physically moving against your problem and into your miracle.

I recently heard of a quadriplegic who could not move any part of his body below his neck. A famous minister laid hands on him for healing and said: keep trying to do something you cannot now do. By the time the man got home he found he could slightly move one finger. He kept doing so until he had full movement in that finger. Then he tried the next finger. He kept up these faith confessions and actions until one year later, he stepped out of his wheelchair. Hallelujah.

If you can only discern a partial relief of your symptoms, you must receive your whole healing, by faith. According to Mark 16:18b, you are in "recovery". Just as the Lord did not quit until the blind man, who saw men as trees walking, was completely healed, He has not sacrificed and triumphed for you to receive only a partial healing.

On the one occasion when Jesus had to pray twice (for the healing of the blind man in Mark 8:22-25), He demonstrated that He would keep on healing the person until the healing was complete and permanent.

Therefore, thank the Lord for both the improvement in your body and for your full healing. Thank God for this promise in His Word.

> *being confident of this, that He Who began a good work in you will carry it on to completion ...*
>
> *Philippians 1:6 NIV*

Command your body to be completely well. Rebuke all symptoms and sickness in Jesus' Name.

Keep thanking the Lord, confessing His Word for your complete healing and commanding your body to be well until you are demonstrating full healing in your body.

In recent years as the worldwide prayer movement has been established by the Lord, two aspects of soaking have been given to the church. Soaking worship is where we praise and wait on God, beholding His Glory by faith, and receive life-changing personal and ministerial impartations and revelations. Soaking prayer is where a person gives or receives prayer over an extended period of time. It may be hours at one time or smaller individual time frames over a long period, even up to a year.

I remember reading a testimony in the first chapter of Dutch Sheets' amazing book (surely one of the best ever written on the topic) "Intercessory Prayer". He visited a comatose lady, whom he calls Diane, many times over the course of a year. When her healing became manifest, after lots of seemingly hopeless diagnoses and situations, the doctors called it a medical miracle. The local newspaper headlined her healing with these words: "Woman Awake, Alive, Healthy After Two Years in a Coma."

My favourite characteristic of our God is His Faithfulness. (refer Hebrews 10:23; 2 Thessalonians 3:3; 1 Corinthians 10:13). We can count on the Lord to fulfil His Word. We can count on the Lord to show up when we need and call upon and believe in Him.

I cannot take Hebrews 6:12 out of the Bible. It says that "faith and patience inherit what has been promised." So, the Lord may test our faith over a period of time, but God will always prove Himself Faithful to His Own Nature, to His Word and to His people.

What to do if you do not discern any physical change?

This is the hardest faith test of all.

There are several instances in the Gospels of people who had no signs of improvement as they left Jesus. This includes (a) those who came to Jesus on behalf of the centurion's servant (Luke 7:1–10); (b) the nobleman whose son was sick in Capernaum (John 4:46–54); (c) the 10 lepers (Luke 17:11–19) and (d) the Syrophonecian mother. (Matthew 15:22–28).

They all had to go on their way in faith, thanking God for the word of healing Jesus gave them and for work of healing they believed would surely come, before any physical change was manifest to them. I am sure they went on their way praising God like Mary did in her beautiful poetic prayer in Luke 1:46–50. They would have said in their hearts and with their mouths what Mary said to the Angel Gabriel: "I am the Lord's servant; be it done to me according to your word." They would have said: "Praise God, when I get there, all will be well."

If they had departed saying "Oh well, I hope something has happened by the time I get home"; or "why didn't Jesus do it right here and now?"; or "this test of faith is too much for me", they could have prevented their miracle from coming into reality. God's Word must be combined with faith in order to produce miracles of answered prayer and fulfilled promises. (Hebrews 4:2).

Peter's falling from faith to fear nearly lost him his life out there on the stormy sea, as well as stopping his miracle in the middle of its realisation. (Matthew 14:22–33). The lesson Peter taught us is this: *We must exercise faith before we receive ministry, while we receive ministry and after we receive ministry.*

I have heard lots of testimonies of people who improved throughout the day, after being ministered to in the morning. Similarly, others have been healed during the night after ministry. Others recover over a week or so. One day they realise, "I am not in pain" or "I am doing what I couldn't do before".

We must choose to believe that every time we receive laying on of hands for healing Divine power flows into our spirit and it will manifest physically.

A word of caution: **Do not stop taking your medication "in faith".** When you are healed, your doctor will confirm it, which will glorify God, and he will tell you the medication is no longer required.

Let me answer this question: Is it OK to receive prayer more than once?

The answer is: of course it's OK.

Jesus taught us to ask and keep on asking; to seek and keep on seeking; to knock and keep on knocking. (Matthew 7:7 NLT). Get prayer as often as you like. BUT, make sure you receive that prayer in faith and both act and speak in faith during and after it.

When Jesus said ask and you will receive, He used a strong word, a military word to describe our receiving. The Greek word "lambano" means "to take" and "to seize". This is not a passive word. To receive the "lambano" way does not wait for God to drop a miracle in your lap. It means pursue your miracle with military determination to enforce Christ's victory over your enemy the devil and over the sickness and the symptoms. Remember, under the terms of the New Testament Covenant, all sickness is from the devil. (Acts 10:38).

What is one thing you have learned from this teaching?

What is one thing you can do to implement this teaching?

Faith Declaration:

I praise You Lord for Your faithfulness and power to make real on earth what is real in Heaven. Your word says You are faithful to do what You have purposed. (1 Thessalonians 5:24). I thank God for what I have already experienced as manifest in my body. By faith, I receive my healing in full, because Jesus did a complete job of purchasing my healing. He does not need to be punished any more for my peace, including my healing. By His wounds I am completely healed. I command my body to be completely well and every symptom of sickness, weakness and dysfunction to cease now and never return, in Jesus' Name. Amen.

14 How to keep your healing

Testimony

As I write this I am waiting for a set of before-and-after medical X-rays that I have been promised. When I prayed, with laying on of hands, for Ps. Elaine in South Australia, all the pain that had discomforted her and restricted her life for a long time left her body. A couple of months of pain-free living later, she went to Royal Adelaide hospital and was told what she already knew: the vertebrae in her back had moved (that is they had been moved by Holy Spirit) into their proper position. She no longer had a back problem that needed treatment.

(1) Don't let the enemy steal what God has given you. After the miracle healing at the pool of Bethesda, Jesus told the lame man who was healed after 38 years of to "go and sin no more, because something worse" could come upon him. So, during and after your healing, you

must live a righteous life for the glory of God. Remember, SIN lets the devil in!

> [21] *Dear friends, if our hearts do not condemn us, we have confidence before God* [22] *and receive from him anything we ask, because we keep his commands and do what pleases him.*
>
> *1 John 3:21–22 NIV*

(2) In John 10:10 Jesus warned us that the devil will try to steal or prevent our healing. James 4:7 tells us to resist the devil until he flees from us. It also says that we must firstly be submitted to God. No one can successfully resist both God and the devil at the same time. Submitting to God means we are obedient to God, to His Word, to His Holy Spirit and to the delegated authorities He has placed in our lives, such as parents, church leaders, employers and government representatives. Like the early apostles said in Acts 5:29, we obey these overseers unless they are asking us to do what is unacceptable to God and contradictory to His Word.

(3) Rebuke the return of any pain (or other symptom). My wife Lynne had pain in a tooth after dental treatment. She continued to command it to stop and the tooth to function normally and painlessly. It did. A young girl broke her leg in an accident at our church one Sunday morning. This was attested to by the mothers of the two

children involved; both mothers were nurses. A few minutes after I prayed for her, she and her mother both walked out of the church and drove home. On the Tuesday, the pain returned. The mother said: Jesus healed you on Sunday, so we are not going to receive this. They rebuked the pain and stood in faith for her ongoing healing in Jesus' Name. The pain left and never returned. She maintained her healing. As I understand it, she was also healed of a mild form of soft bone syndrome that had caused her to have various sprains and breaks during her early childhood. Glory to God. Command your body to be well and all symptoms of sickness to stop, that is, to go and stay gone. Take authority over the spirit of pain and the spirit of infirmity in Jesus' Name. Command them to flee and never return.

(4) 3 John 2 tells us that a healthy soul is necessary for our bodies to be healthy. So, keep your heart and mind free of things like hurts, offences, un-forgiveness, resentments, jealousy, anger, prejudice and judgementalism. This helps you to receive what the Lord Jesus Christ has done for you. It doesn't prevent God from healing you unconditionally, but three reasons Jesus couldn't heal in his own home town were lack of honour; offence; and unbelief, which is the wilful refusal to believe. Period.

(5) Pray for others to be healed, both in intercession and in ministry when you lay hands on the sick for their

healing. When Job prayed for his friends he received the double portion in every area of life, including his own healing. (Job 42:10).

(6) Keep speaking the healing promises of God over your body, life and ministry. Mrs. Dodie Osteen has a stunning testimony of her healing from cancer. She quoted the healing Scriptures day and night until she was healed. Thirty plus years of good health later, she still quotes them daily. Ps. Dodie also pushed herself to go and pray for others even when she was not feeling well herself. These faith actions produced the reward of healing from the cancer and decades of good health.

(7) Keep remembering the benefits of your full salvation (Psalm 103:1-5) and the character and power of our God. He is your committed Covenant Healer and the Lord to Whom nothing and no one are impossible. He is El Shaddai, the All-Mighty God of Miracles and the God of Plenty. The Lord will not fail you, forsake you, nor forget you. He is on your side and by your side always. God is good and He only does good. He delights to do you good and to give you good gifts. The Lord has brought you into His family with the twin guarantees of Holy Spirit's indwelling presence and the better promises of the better new Covenant. God will never afflict you with sickness, from which He sent Jesus to the Cross to deliver you. Our Heavenly Father, our Saviour, Lord and Shepherd, our Paraclete and Helper, the wonderful,

powerful Triune God Whom we worship and serve will never hurt or harm us. He is committed to helping and healing us. Hallelujah.

What is one thing you have learned from this teaching?

What is one thing you can do to implement this teaching?

Faith Declaration:

I praise You Lord because, as Abraham proved by having more children through Keturah (Genesis 25:1), what You heal stays healed. I praise Jesus for what He has done for me. I rejoice in Your goodness, greatness and grace toward me and all people. I thank You Lord for my manifest healing. I thank You for my complete and permanent healing. I command my body to stay well and the devil to flee from me and stay gone in Jesus' name. Amen.

15 Minister healing as Jesus did

Testimony

Raphael gave me his video testimony after his healings in Orlando, Florida, USA. He said he came to church in "terrible, terrible pain". It was caused by three herniated discs and a damaged Achilles tendon. Holy Spirit quickened his body as he released his faith during the prayer ministry time. He said all the pain from those conditions left him. Then he said he had a third problem, namely a stabbing pain in his left leg. He felt that leg start to shake and then it was as if he heard a "pop". All the pain was gone. He had a night of peace and was completely healed and pain free, as he testified to me the day after he received his healings.

I want to share with you a way to pray that the Lord Himself revealed to me. It helped me understand how Jesus ministered and how He taught the disciples in the early church to do the same.

As I have used this method around the world, people have been healed of many physical needs, especially from painful conditions including necks, shoulders, hands, hips, backs, knees and ankles.

There were two things that puzzled me, because they seemed to be contradictory to each other.

Firstly, I noticed that when Jesus healed the sick, He always commanded the person to be healed or delivered of a demon. Jesus never asked God to heal or deliver them.

Secondly, I knew there were plenty of Scriptures about prayer, and some of my favourites were about asking God to do things, with the expectation that He would answer and therefore we would receive what we asked for.

So what are we to do ?

Do we *ask* God for Healing?

or

Do we *command* Healing to happen?

The answer is: we are to do both.

Many times Jesus went away on His Own to pray. This is when He asked the Father to heal the sick.

After Jesus had asked the Father to heal the sick through Him, Jesus then acted in faith, by commanding the healings He had prayed for to happen. Jesus acted in faith, as if He knew that the Father had answered His prayer.

I believe Jesus was practicing what he preached in the Gospel of Matthew.

> *But when you pray, go into your room, close the door and pray to your Father, who is unseen. Then your Father, who sees what is done in secret, will reward you.*
> *Matthew 6:6 NIV*

After you pray in private, God will reward you with results when you minister in public.

So, the way we minister like Jesus did is this:

- We privately ask the Father to heal the sick, in Jesus Name
- We believe it is the Father's Will to heal the sick, because the Bible teaches us this is true.
- We believe the Father has heard and granted our Prayer (1 John 5:14–15).
- We publicly act as if the Father has heard and granted our prayer. We do this by commanding healings to take place, in Jesus' Name, when we minister to people. Commanding is how Jesus ministered to people in every recorded instance of His many healings,

deliverances and miracles in the Gospels. The same principle is taught by this saying: Don't speak about your mountain, speak to your mountain. By faith, you command it to depart from your life or that of the person to whom you are ministering.

- Similarly, don't speak about how big or threatening the storm is. The only way to still that storm is by commanding it to stop affecting your life, in Jesus' Name.

However there are two other considerations to be added into our ministry preparations.

The first is the recognition of the importance of thanksgiving, praise and worship.

> *Do not be anxious or worried about anything, but in everything [every circumstance and situation] by prayer and petition with thanksgiving, continue to make your [specific] requests known to God.*
>
> *Philippians 4:6*
>
> *He who sacrifices thank offerings honours me, and he prepares the way so that I may show (literally: make visible) him the salvation of God."*
> *Psalm 50:23 NIV (2009)*

When we thank God for Who He is and for what He has done and for what we have already received and for what He has promised to give us, we prepare the way spiritually for the Lord to give us more of His salvation blessings and benefits.

When we spend worship and waiting time in His Presence, we are touched, changed and empowered. (2 Corinthians 3:18). Just as Jesus did, we go into the secret, personal, intimate place of communion with God for relationship and for the infilling of Holy Spirit. Then, we take His Presence, Power and Glory out into our world to give away to others.

The second consideration is that of persistence in prayer (asking); persistence in the Word of God (seeking. I once had the Lord say to me "Seek Me in My Word" – John 5:39) and persistence in ministry (knocking, or acting in faith).

> *Because everyone who keeps asking will receive, and the person who keeps searching will find, and the person who keeps knocking will have the door opened.*
>
> *Matthew 7:8 ISV*

This now leads me to the acronym (T–A–C–K) that the Lord revealed me so that we learn to minister as Jesus did.

T is for Thanksgiving, Praise and Worship

A is for Asking God for healing in prayer

C is for Commanding healing to manifest when you are in the time of ministry

K is to Keep on Thanking, Asking and Commanding until the answer has fully manifested.

Let me finish with a classic example from the Scriptures of how the apostle Peter put this method into practice, resulting in a miracle – the raising of Dorcas.

> *Peter sent them all out of the room; then he got down on his knees and prayed. Turning toward the dead woman, he said, "Tabitha, get up." She opened her eyes, and seeing Peter she sat up.*
>
> *Acts 9:40*

Peter first did something he had seen Jesus do – he sent all the grieving people, who had no faith for a miracle, out of the room.

Then, Peter turned away from the body, so as to focus on the Lord. This is a good thing to do. Don't let your symptoms or someone's long description of their problems rob you of faith. Turn to God, for Whom all things are possible.

While Acts does not tell us exactly how Peter prayed, I am sure you understand that he would have quieted himself before God; thanked the Lord for His miracle working power; and asked the Lord to do again through Peter, what He did through Jesus and do it for the glory of God, as well as for the benefit of Dorcas and her family and friends. This is the "T" and "A" in "T-A-C-K".

Having asked for a fresh infilling of Holy Spirit (such as he received in Acts 4:8a) and for a miracle of healing and resurrection, Peter then turned to the body and commanded her to "get up". This is the "C" in "T-A-C-K".

Dorcas woke up healed and alive and Peter helped her get to her feet. Then he presented her alive to the people. This resulted in "many people" believing in the Lord.

There is no record here in Acts 9 of Peter having to pray or command more than once. So, in this case he did not need to **keep on** thanking, asking and commanding.

However, from my own experience I know Peter didn't ask only at this one time for miracles to happen. He was constantly asking, confessing, believing and acting in faith for such miracles to accredit his ministry as they did Jesus. (Acts 2:22; John 14:11).

I have asked the Lord many times over the years for the spiritual gift of healing pain and all its causes. Praise God He has given it to me. For this I say: "Thanks God" and "More, Lord."

There are times – too many for my liking – when just as Jesus prayed a second time for a blind man to be completely healed, we have to pray more than once for a person's healing to be fully manifested. A lot of people only receive a partial healing after one faith command. Pushing into God for the fulfilling of that healing requires faith. One of the reasons the spiritual gift of "working of miracles" was given that name is because it can take persistence for a person to minister a miracle to someone and persistence for the person to receive their healing in full. This is another aspect of what I mean by the "K" in "T-A-C-K".

I cannot over-emphasise the spiritual power of God that is released by speaking Bible-based words in faith. (Proverbs 12:14; Proverbs 18:20-21). It is certainly a faith action when you rebuke a fever as Jesus did in Luke 4:39. The result in that instance was the healing of Peter's mother in law.

It takes faith to command pain to go, symptoms to stop, demons to flee and healing to manifest now! When you do speak such faith commands in the Name of Jesus – the Name above all names including "pain" – miracles can, do and must happen.

It takes faith for the weak to say: "I am strong." (Joel 3:10).

It is also important to not say negative things that are not in accord with God's Word. (eg Jeremiah 1:7)

What is one thing you have learned from this teaching?

____

What is one thing you can do to implement this teaching?

____

Faith Declaration:

I thank You Lord for enabling every willing believer in Jesus and Your Word to have a healing ministry. I praise You for giving us access to Your Presence and Power. I ask You for the spiritual gifts of healing, faith and the working of miracles. I speak into being in Jesus' Name that as I lay hands on the sick they will recover. I ask for and declare in Jesus' Name that all symptoms, including pain, will leave as their conditions are healed completely and permanently. I ask for and believe to be used in all kinds of healings, such as eyes, ears, skin, auto-immune problems, skeletal and dental needs and for the healing of people's chronic needs. I declare that as I step out in faith, You Lord will back me up and show up to manifest the works and glory of God, according to 2 Thessalonians 1:11-12. I pray all these healings will be for His glory and lead to many people believing in and following Jesus as a lifestyle. Amen

16 Healing mysteries and medical help

Testimony

The ministry time in Belfast City church, Northern Ireland, was awesome. There were plenty of healing testimonies, including several who said that when I commanded pain to go, it went. An African lady demonstrated her healing from a bad knee she had endured for years. Another woman's shoulder problem, which she also had put up with for years, was healed and she had freedom of movement. Doreen from Antrim was healed of neck and shoulder pain and stiffness. A retired pastor received a "spot-on" prophecy and was healed of both shoulder pain and restricted movement.

Grief from Death of a Loved One

> *.... all the days ordained for me were written in your book before one of them came to be.*
> *Psalm 139:16*

> *The Lord is my shepherd,*
> *I shall not want. Even though I walk through the valley of the shadow of death, I fear no evil, for You are with me; Your rod and Your staff, they comfort me.*
> *Psalm 23:1,4*

Let me begin by saying it is okay to feel grief and pain when we lose a loved one. It is okay to grieve. We know from the New Testament that there were times when Jesus grieved. It is not a weakness. It is not a sin.

Jesus said, "Blessed are those who mourn" God's grace is sufficient for all situations and seasons, no matter how long they last. God promises to give us beauty for ashes, the Oil of Joy for mourning. Keep believing for the evidence of His Divine partnership in your life.

Sadly, we humans are not yet immortal, although one day, according to 1 Corinthians 15:53-58, we will be. The shadow of people dear to us who die, does pass over us. In such times, when we feel we have been unwillingly dragged into a valley of grief, depression, shock, numbness, loneliness, fear and even anger, the Lord is with us to help us get through our grief and loss and to go forward again in life.

These feelings are increased when a parent has to bury a child (of any age). The Lord's presence is also increased, because He gives grace that is sufficient for every need.

The worst grief I felt was when my grandson Andrew died in my daughter's womb not long before he was due to be born. It was as if I was in a fog for six months. I honestly do not know how I got through that period. I can only say: Thank You Lord that I did.

I often think of how even the Father lost His Son, Jesus, at an early age. That encourages me to know that God understands what we are going through. He helps us according to our needs .... and according to our willingness to allow Him to help.

The timing of any person's death cannot be predicted, nor understood. In the end, I believe the matter of the timing of death is in God's Hands alone, not man's and not the devil's.

We must believe that the Lord is perfect in character and never makes a mistake, nor does anything wrong (Deuteronomy 32:4). If we blame Him for the problem, how can we also look to Him in faith as our Answer?

I give my sincere condolences to those who have experienced grief and to those who are going through that valley now. I pray you will know the Presence, peace, power, protection and provision of the Lord your Shepherd with you day and night.

We must leave with God the spiritual status of those who have died. It is not for us to judge. I encourage you to pray with me the prayer Holy Spirit gave me to share with others. Ask God to save people in their last day on earth, or their last 24 days or weeks. I believe the Lord showed me that many thousands upon thousands will be saved through this prayer.

I believe God's mercy is so oceanic and His grace so overwhelming and the sacrifice and triumph of Jesus so important, that all He requires is a simple "help, Lord" in the last seconds of a person's life, in order for Him to open His saving arms to them.

Disabilities, Suffering, Persecution and Trouble

> *These things I have spoken to you, so that in Me you may have peace. In the world you have tribulation, but take courage; I have overcome the world.*
>
> *John 16:33 NASB*

Other translations of this verse say that while we are living in this world, we shall experience "troubles, trials, sorrows, suffering, oppression, distress and/or affliction."

We have probably all heard the saying: "You can't have a testimony without a test."

> *6 In this you greatly rejoice, even though now for a little while, if necessary, you have been distressed by various trials, 7 so that the proof of your faith, being more precious than gold which is perishable, even though tested by fire, may be found to result in praise and glory and honour at the revelation of Jesus Christ;*
>
> *1 Peter 1:6-7*

Life, circumstances, people and the devil have ways of throwing hurdles in our way and placing heavy burdens upon us. The Bible promises Christians that we shall not be tested beyond what we can bear. (1 Corinthians 10:13). So, even when our faith is being tested, stretched, proven, we can look to Jesus, our Emmanuel, God-with-us, to get us through. As we put our faith in Him and the Word of God, we will find that we can "do all things through Christ Who strengthens us." (Philippians 4:13). I have been in seasons where I felt I could not go even another step forward; but God has empowered me to go another mile.

We all have to deal with problems and pressures. Unfortunately some people may have to deal with far more than others. There are those who seem able to endure levels of pressure that are breathtakingly courageous. I believe God gives us grace to handle situations as they arise. We must prepare for tough times before they come. When they come God releases His grace to get us through.

I want to acknowledge here especially those carers who have family members with disabilities. Sometimes the carer is a child and the one in need is a parent. There are cases where siblings lose their parents while they are young. Some of the older siblings act as parents to their younger brothers and sisters.

People who are in circumstances of life like these deserve special recognition and support and reward. They and the pastors, leaders and members of churches, human rights organisations and charities, the health and social work vocations, counsellors and special-education teachers are heroes in society.

The Bible indicates that God is closest to those whose life is the toughest (Psalm 34: 18-19) and that His grace will always be sufficient. (2 Corinthians 12:9). I pray His presence, peace, power and provision are evident in each and every such life. May God, as El Shaddai, the Lord All-Mighty, Who is more-than-enough, meet every need for life and godliness, in abundance and far above all these people can ask or think, in Jesus' Name. Amen.

The Bible says we Christians should remember the poor, the sick, the imprisoned, the persecuted and the oppressed. If all we can do is pray, then let us pray. If we can do more, such as give or serve, then let us do so as unto the Lord. (Matthew 25:34-46; Galatians 6:2).

If you are going through hard to bear circumstances, either temporarily or as a lifestyle, please do not bear it alone. Seek Christian, governmental, charitable and professional help. Let another believer be "God-with-skin-on" to you. Again, this is the central point of James 5:14-16; do not be sick or unhappy alone. Call for the help of Christ's body, the church.

Some people don't get healed

There are things about Divine Healing that cannot be explained. I can't tell you why Paul, the greatest miracle-worker in the early church, had to leave Trophimus sick in Miletus. (2 Timothy 4:20).

We are also told that Epaphroditus was very sick indeed, possibly due to overwork. (Philippians 2:25-30). So, we should exercise wisdom as well as faith in the matter of Divine healing and the even better benefit of the Christian Gospel, namely, walking in Divine health.

Most healing ministers will have stories of people who did not get healed and even of some who died. Jesus is the only One I know who had a 100% record of healing everyone He ministered to. The Gospels report 17 times that Jesus healed everyone present which, because of some doubling up of the Gospel narratives, is actually 12 separate occasions. On two of those occasions, namely the feeding of the 5,000 (Matthew 14:14) and the 4,000 (Matthew 15:30-31), there were literally thousands present.

The choice you have to make (and "faith" is simply "making a Biblical choice") is whether you will focus on the plain teachings of Jesus' ministry in the Gospels or on the negative experiences and/or scepticism of others.

The fact that somebody in the Bible or in your life experience did not get healed, either the first time they were prayed for, or the twentieth time, or not at all, does not change the Word or Nature or Ways of God.

Our faith must be based on God's Word alone and, in regard to Divine healing, our faith must be Christo-centric, New Covenant faith.

The plain teaching of the Gospels is that anyone can be healed anytime, just by going to Jesus and asking for their healing. He always gave it unconditionally and immediately. Our faith should be for nothing less than that.

I cannot explain why some people are healed and others are not. I certainly do not believe God picks and chooses whom He will heal because salvation, including healing, is available to anyone and everyone. Jesus never refused a single person who came to Him for healing. He resisted but did not refuse to give His power to even an unqualified person, which is how He described the Syrophonecian mother.

I do not believe in blaming the patient for a lack of faith. I would more quickly challenge myself to have more faith as a minister of healing to others, in Jesus' Name.

I must tell you that the teaching in James 5:14-16 concerning confessing our sins and faults and mistakes before we receive healing *does not mean that every illness has a corresponding sin.* Jesus made this clear in John 9:1-3. So, we should ***never say*** to a person who is having difficulty receiving their healing: *"You must have* *sin in your life."* Rather examine our own hearts to see if we are falling short of the grace of God in some way. (Matthew 7:3–5).

The word "if" in James 5:15 does indicate the possibility that the illness might have been induced by, and the devil invited in by, some unconfessed (and unrepented of) sin in the person's life. That is one of the reasons James wrote those verses, so the sick would repent if sin was a stumbling block to their healing.

Sickness may occasionally be the fruit of sin, but it is not often a sign of sin. Most Christians who are sick do not have unconfessed sin in their lives. They may have stress, but not sin.

So, beware of any doctrine or preacher who teaches sickness is a sign of sin or of a lack of faith. There are many healthy sinners and unbelievers in our world. Why they are not all sick is a mystery to people who blame sin in the sick person's life for their current lack of healing.

There are many complicating and intersecting factors involved in the Divine healing of our physical conditions. In the end we just have to keep our faith in God and His Word and in what Jesus has done for us, until we are healed and then after we are healed.

The real decision you need to make in regard to healing is to get your mind off everything except the Lord Jesus and the Word of God. Don't focus on sad stories; religious theologies; things that your mind is never going to understand; demonic doubts, fears and unbelief; symptoms and/or what the internet says about them; or medical scepticism concerning the Lord. Start every day as a new day of hope and healing.

God does not use sickness as a faith-testing or teaching tool

There is no Biblical teaching in the New Covenant age of Grace that says God afflicts His people with sickness to test their faith, nor that He uses sickness to teach His people something.

God is glorified by healing, not by sickness. Over and over the Bible makes it clear that Satan is the author of sickness, as was the case with Job (Job 2:7) and the woman the devil had bound for eighteen years. (Luke 13:16).

In the raising of Lazarus, God was glorified by his healing and resurrection, not by his sickness and death. (John 11:4). Similarly, the healing of the blind man was what demonstrated the works of God, not his blindness. (John 9:3).

God does not afflict His people with sickness to make them more like Christ or more obedient.

Although there are glowing exceptions to this, the normal fact of the matter is that most people are worse Christians when they are sick, not better ones. They hardly pray. They don't read their Bibles much. They don't serve anyone else. They are negative, not positive

.... until they are well again. Then, they get on with their lives and ministries.

The three primary instruments of teaching that God uses are: (i) His Word; (ii) His Spirit; and (iii) His anointed, experienced, mature-in-Christ-and-in-God's-Word people, who teach us personally or indirectly through their books, CD's, YouTube videos, TV programs, podcasts, testimonies etc.

Of course, we also learn from our own experiences, meaning our good and bad decisions and their consequences, and from that of others.

God disciplines Christians, but never punishes us

It is important to understand that God punished Jesus for us. Therefore God cannot punish us, because Jesus has already taken our punishment upon Himself.

There are two different Greek words that are used for "punishment" (1 John 4:18 "kolasin", meaning "penal infliction") and "discipline"
(Hebrews 12:10 "paideuo", meaning "chasten, correct, train, educate").

My understanding of how God disciplines us is that He uses a progressive plan:

(1) God "goads" us, as He did Paul. (Acts 26:14). He annoys our conscience by His Word and by His Spirit.

(2) He goes Silent, like a teacher in a noisy classroom. He withdraws His Voice.

(3) He withdraws His power. Life gets tough. We realise that we are doing things in our own strength. Our circumstances become adverse. Proverbs 13:15 says: the way of the transgressor is hard. Our heart may now start getting hard against God. We get resentful of His lack of evidence in our lives. So, our life gets harder, because the principle of 3 John 2 works in the negative, as well as the positive. If my soul is not prospering, my life will not prosper.

(4) God seems to be Absent. He withdraws His Presence. God hides Himself. (Isaiah 45:15). He wants us to hunger for Him and cry out to Him, as David did in Psalm 51: 11 and 12.

> *11 "Do not cast me from your presence or take your Holy Spirit from me. 12 Restore to me the joy of your salvation and grant me a willing spirit, to sustain me."*

(5) We realise we are getting stressed and/or negative OR others realise we are stressed and negative

(6) God disciplines us through other people, especially family members, close friends or leaders.

(7) We get so out of touch with God and so deep into the world's and the devil's sphere of influence that our faith to receive God's blessing, including healing, is at an

all-time low. We are most vulnerable to the attacks of our enemy the devil, who certainly does use sickness against us. Jesus treated all sickness as a curse from Satan, not a blessing from God. We are now in danger of what is described in Paul's famous Communion passage. (1 Corinthians 11:29,30). Christians can get weak, sick or even die, through self-condemnation, self-inflicted punishment, not taking care of themselves, or accepting ill-treatment from others, because they feel they deserve it. When we consider the parable of the unforgiving debtor in Matthew 18:34,35, we learn that the tormenting jailers are demons, but some people wrongly think it's God, who is making their lives miserable. This is a dangerous time, when the temptation to self-medicate the bad feelings is strong. Such actions make the person feel worse, not better, and may lead to very harmful life situations.

(8) The final step is that we can infect other people in our lives with these negative things. Our stubbornness, anger, depression, or bitterness begins to defile others. (Hebrews 12:15). Then things really turn sour, because they start rejecting us, blaming us, or worse still, joining us in the darkness we are wallowing in. By this stage, people can get very isolated and either suicidally depressed or rebelliously disobedient to God and to everyone who is trying to help them. Consequentially, life goes from hard to harder (refer Proverbs 13:15 KJB).

I urge any who are at this stage of the Lord's discipline to humble yourselves, admit where you are at and get the help you need, especially from the Lord, His Word and His people.

> *No discipline seems pleasant at the time, but painful. Later on, however, it produces a harvest of righteousness and peace for those who have been trained by it.*
> *Hebrews 12:11*

Is there a specific time for a person to be healed?

My reply is that God's time is now, because He is the great "I AM", the God of the now. One of the challenges of our faith is to believe, according to Matthew 18:20, Jesus, the Lord Who heals us, is in the room with us NOW.

> *Let us then approach God's throne of grace with confidence, so that we may receive mercy and find grace to help us in our time of need.*
>
> *Hebrews 4:16 NIV*

The NLT says "when we need it most."

The Amplified Bible reads "find [His amazing] grace to help in time of need [an appropriate blessing, coming just at the right moment]."

If you do not believe for healing now, you will be constantly frustrated by a healing you do not receive, because you are not believing to receive it yet.

However, we do know God has a timetable for things such as the End Times, just as He had for the birth of Jesus. But does He have a timetable for every single healing that takes place on earth?

My theology is that God foreknows everything, but does not fore-ordain everything. I cannot explain this fully here in this chapter.

In Jesus' ministry, He was often moved to do healings and miracles by what seemed to be "interruptions", not scheduled appointments. Examples of this are the healings of Jairus' daughter (Matthew 9:18–26) and the servant of the centurion (Luke 7:1–10) and the Nobleman's son. (John 4:46–54).

Could we say the healing of the man at the Gate Beautiful was an appointed time? Had Jesus walked past him on previous occasions? Did Jesus not heal him because it wasn't his time to be healed until Peter and John walked past him that wonderful day?

I think that if there really was a specifically appointed time for everyone to be healed, we would see in the Gospel records that of the many thousands of people He healed, there would have been some instances where Jesus said to various people: "It's not your time to be healed today."

Rather than say "it's not your time" to even one person in a village or crowd, the Bible says Jesus healed "all". (Acts 10:38). There are 17 Gospel passages that directly say or imply that Jesus healed "all" who were in His Presence.

- 9 references in Matthew

4:23–24; 8:16–17; 9:35; 12:15; 14:14; 14:34–36; 15:30–31; 19:2; 21:14

- 3 references in Mark

1:32–34; 1:39; 6:56

- 5 references in Luke

4:40; 6:17–19; 7:21; 9:11; 17:12–17

These represent literally thousands of healings without a single mention of anyone having to wait for a specific time.

Similarly, when Jesus commissioned His followers to go out and preach the Kingdom, with power to heal the sick and authority to cast out demons, He never gave them instruction to be careful not to heal anyone before it was God's time for their healing. (Matthew 10:1 & 8; Mark 16:15–20; Luke 9:1–2; Luke 10: 1 & 9).

> *For everything there is a season, and a time for every matter under heaven*
>
> *Ecclesiastes 11:1 ESV*

I could still say of this verse that the time for healing is now, not some other unknown calendar date.

Both Young's Literal translation and Darby Bible Translation end Hebrews 4:16 this way: "find grace for seasonable help." So, they would agree with me that the time for healing is in the season when you need to be healed.

I believe there is Biblical authority for Christians to be able to change, by faith, any specific divine timetable, to our own "now". I have several reasons for saying this:

- Matthew 24:20 says we can pray that something will not happen in winter, nor on a Sabbath. This means our prayers and faith can influence God's Timetable.

- The woman with the issue of blood, by her own faith initiative, set her own time and method to be healed. (Mark 5:28). Jesus had no idea who touched Him. Jesus did not choose to heal her, she chose to be healed by Him. Jesus did not choose when to heal her, she did.

- At the wedding in Cana, Jesus told Mary: "My hour has not yet come." Mary then told the servants in faith "Do whatever He tells you." Then Jesus did the miracle of turning the water into wine. Mary's faith had pulled a miracle out of the future into the now. Another way of saying it is that Mary's faith moved God to do something that even Jesus did not know was about to happen.

- The Syrophoenician-Canaanite mother similarly overcame Jesus' reluctance and by faith chose the timing of her daughter's healing miracle. (Matthew 15:21-28).

Medical and Dental Help

I need to make my full position clear. You might ask: "Does Nick believe in receiving treatment from doctors and dentists?" My answer is: "Yes."

I believe medical science is one aspect of the fulfilling of the prophecy in Daniel (12:4) re the "increase of knowledge". I believe the "sick need a physician" as Jesus Himself said in Mark 2:17.

This is illustrated in the Old Testament by King Hezekiah's healing in Isaiah 38:21.

Timothy was encouraged to use a little wine for his stomach and frequent ailments. (1 Timothy 5:23). This is like using wisdom as well as faith for his health's sake. Mature Christians know that faith and wisdom are brothers, not enemies. However, do not use "wisdom" as an excuse for unbelief.

I believe in having both faith for God's Divine healing and wisdom to pursue the best medical advice and treatment that doctors and dentists can provide.

The glory will always go to the Lord for our improvement and full restoration, because, as one doctor is reported to have said: We treat our patients, but it is God Who heals.

This is in accord with the Bible's revelation that God gave Himself the Name "Jehovah Rapha", which means: "I am the Lord Who heals you."

The Lord has committed Himself in a covenant way to helping us get well when we are sick. Hallelujah.

My goal in this book is to inspire you to believe God to both receive Divine healing and impart it to others. I do not want believers to be limited to medical science, nor to a "che sera sera" approach, which fatalistically represents thinking that "whatever will be, will be." Jesus purchased Divine healing for all. Christians should put prayer before painkillers. We should seek God first for our healing, before we turn to doctors.

I repeat my word of caution: **Do not stop taking your medication "in faith".** When you are healed, your doctor will confirm it, which will glorify God, and he will tell you the medication is no longer required.

Conclusion

This is a quote from my book "Holy Spirit Faith Food Snack Pack", chapter 4, pages 65-66.

Anyone who believes in Jesus and in the Word of God is equally able and qualified in Christ to receive both the forgiveness of their sins and the healing of their bodies. The sacrifice of Jesus made both forgiveness and healing available to us. We do not earn, deserve or self-qualify for these blessings. God gives them freely to us in honour of His Son, Jesus. They can only be claimed by faith.

It is important for me to emphasise that just as we cannot earn our forgiveness and our place in God's heaven, so we cannot earn our healing.

The wonderful good news of the Christian Gospel is that all we need to receive God's many blessings that are freely given to us by His grace, is to have faith. We have faith in what Jesus did for each and every one of us.

No-one is more qualified or less qualified to receive healing from Jesus. He was punished so that every person of every nation and every generation could experience His full salvation for spirit, soul, body and life.

You can confidently say – and I urge you to do so out loud right now – "Healing belongs to me because of what Jesus did for me."

Many people readily accept the benefit of God's forgiveness of their sins, but fail to accept the benefit of healing for their bodies. This is partly due to the lack of preaching about healing as being included in our salvation.

Many pastors preach only part of the Gospel, the spiritual part, the "eternal life" part, which is about the forgiveness of our sins. Sadly, they ignore the natural blessings and benefits that Jesus has also made available to us – the "abundant life" aspects of salvation. The natural part of the Gospel includes healing for the mind and the body and provision for life and ministry.

For the purposes of this chapter, my key point is that whenever and wherever the "full Gospel" is preached, healing for the body is included.

My final thought is this. My goal in writing this book is to inspire you to build and activate your faith firstly to receive your healing and secondly, to develop your healing ministry to other people. To that end I pray God will anoint you richly, reveal Himself to you in His Word and by His Spirit and give you great encouragement and success as you step out in faith for yourself and others, in Jesus' Name. Amen.

So now it's up to you to "GO FOR IT!"

What is one thing you have learned from this teaching?

What is one thing you can do to implement this teaching?

Faith Declaration:

I praise You Lord because You are faithful and true and Your word is faithful and true. I thank You for every healing that has taken place since Jesus came to save us. I praise You for having no prejudice for or against anyone. I thank You that Jesus suffered and triumphed for all people. Lord I yield to You my lack of understanding of the mysteries that occur in healing ministry and declare that I trust in You with all my heart. By faith I choose to not focus on negative reports, as the 10 spies did, but to be as Joshua and Caleb and declare the inheritance of healing is ours through Jesus Christ our Lord. (Numbers 13:26-14:9). I declare that God's word is true, no matter what circumstance I am faced with. I declare that His story in God's Word outranks every other story in human history. Lord I praise You for the increase of knowledge that Daniel prophesied has happened in medicine. I give You glory for all successful medical treatment that doctors have given and will give. I ask You to do more both through the medical profession and supernaturally, and declare it will be so, in Jesus' Name. Amen.

ABOUT THE AUTHOR

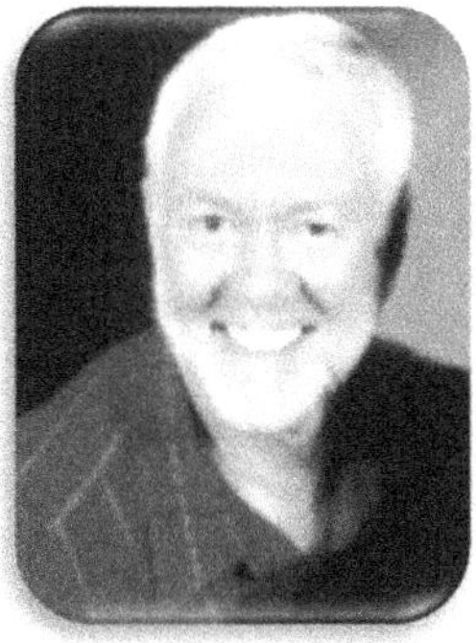

Nick Watson has been happily married to Lynne since 1970. They have 3 children, Kylie, Simon and Rebekah; 4 grandchildren Katie, Rennick, Craig and Aiden; and 1 great-granddaughter, Riley.

Nick is the Founder, Principal Prophet, Author and Teacher, and People Builder of Prophetic Power Ministries.

He was for years the Senior Pastor of Bayside Christian Family (Apostolic) Church, a thriving Spirit-filled church in Brisbane, Queensland. Australia.

Nick has been a recognised prophet in the Apostolic Church Australia for more than 25 years. He has served in various denominational leadership roles.

Nick has preached and prophesied throughout Australia and overseas, with a signs-following ministry.

YOUR FEEDBACK

If this book has encouraged your faith, please share your testimony with us at the email address below.

Contact Nick Watson

If you desire to contact Nick concerning a ministry engagement at your church, group, camp or leaders' event please visit our website:

www.youcanprophesy.com

www.facebook.com/nickjwatson.ycp

GMail

email: youcanprophesy@gmail.com

OTHER BOOKS by Nick Watson

Faith Food Snack Pack – Overcoming

Faith Food Snack Pack – Good News

Faith Food Snack Pack – Healthy Soul

Faith Food Snack Pack – Holy Spirit

34 Faith-Lifters that Bless and Build Believers (this is a compilation of the 4 Snack Packs into one volume.)

You Can Prophesy
Supernatural. Simple. Safe.

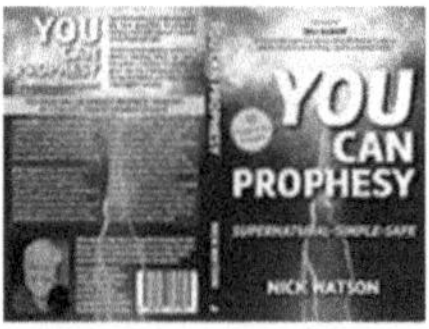

www.ingramcontent.com/pod-product-compliance
Lightning Source LLC
Chambersburg PA
CBHW030244030426
42336CB00009B/249
9780994301253